Catch That Look

Living, Laughing & Loving Despite Triple-Negative Breast Cancer

A Memoir
Ann Pietrangelo

DEDICATION

for those who survive
for those we've lost
for those who love

TABLE OF CONTENTS

FOREWORD

Through my over two-decade career as a breast surgical oncologist, I have seen and treated numerous patients with triple-negative breast cancer. Breast cancers are characterized, in part, by the presence or absence of receptors on the surface of the cancer cells. The presence of hormone receptors – estrogen and progesterone – can predict the responsiveness of the cancer to anti-estrogen drugs. Human epidermal growth factor (HER2) receptor positive cancer can be treated with specific targeted therapy. Triple-negative cancers are negative for estrogen receptor, progesterone receptor, and HER2. Between ten and fifteen percent of all breast cancers in the United States are of the triple negative variety. Such cancers are more likely to occur in younger women, those of African descent, and BRCA1 mutation carriers.

In this wonderful volume, Ann Pietrangelo leads the reader on a journey through her diagnosis and tri-modality treatment – surgery, chemotherapy, and radiation. Her breast cancer diagnosis came seven years after a diagnosis of another life-altering disease – multiple sclerosis. To quote from her first memoir *No More Secs!* she must have felt "like the ball in a pinball machine, bouncing haplessly from bumper to bumper at the mercy of an unseen player." She tells her story of crossing over into cancer land with candor, never losing her sense of humor. This book gives insight not just for patients, but also for their caregivers and loved ones. Breast cancer affects not just the women and men diagnosed with the disease, but the entire family. Ann is blessed to have a loving and supportive family. Her bond with her husband Jim reminds us, as Ann tells us, nothing in life matters as much as love.

Advances in our understanding of the biology and treatment of triple-negative breast cancer (TNBC) occur daily, thanks to those clinicians and scientists dedicated to research and its application to patient care. The recognition that triple-negative cancer occurs more commonly in genetically predisposed women led the National Cooperative Cancer Network to change its guidelines in 2011. Testing for BRCA1 and 2 mutations is now recommended for women diagnosed with TNBC at or below age 60.

I commend Ann for her veracity and tenacity. This book will have lasting value, and I'm glad she chose to share her experiences with us, to teach us all to live, laugh, and love.

Diane Radford MD, FACS, FRCSEd
St. Louis, MO
October 2013

INTRODUCTION

I vowed to myself, and to all who inquired, that I would not write this book. Yet, here it is, a second memoir that involves my own health.

When I wrote *No More Secs! Living, Laughing & Loving Despite Multiple Sclerosis*, my intention was to pull the reader inside the thought process of a person as she comes to grips with a serious health condition.

It worked. I occasionally receive emails from readers of *No More Secs!* Some thank me for writing it and putting into words what they were unable to express. Some say they used it to tell their loved ones what it feels like to have MS. Some tell me they simply feel less alone.

My "living, laughing, and loving despite" mindset worked well enough for multiple sclerosis, but throwing triple-negative breast cancer into the mix would test my resolve, and that of my husband.

Like *No More Secs!*, *Catch That Look* is about more than cancer. It's a love story. Romantic love. Love of family. Love of life. It's about LIVING while you're here.

After the cancer diagnosis, someone attempted to comfort me by saying, "Now you'll have more credibility as a health writer." That's a bit of credibility I could have lived without. Still, if my story provides a small measure of comfort to one person, it's a story worth telling.

CHAPTER 1

Oh, Crap!

Thursday, October 14, 2010. That's the day I accidentally stumbled upon the invader that would so profoundly affect my life. As that most ordinary of days unfolded, I was blissfully unaware of the aggressive cells that were stealthily dividing and invading nearby tissue within my body.

You don't necessarily recognize life-altering events as they happen. After everything changes, you can't help but try to trace back to that ground zero moment when a particular chain of events was set into motion.

I can't trace this chain of events further back than that day, the Day of the Lump, and I will never find that first link. Did it exist even before I was born? Was I exposed to the wrong chemicals in the air I breathe, the food I eat, or the places I've lived and worked? Were there any clues? How could I possibly have felt so good while my would-be assassin was staking claim on my body?

Since the lump is where my awareness of the chain began, I would soon come to think in terms of "before the lump" and "after the lump," and later "Before Cancer" and "After Cancer."

Like everyone on Earth, my life is filled with before and after chapters. Before and after marriage, before and after children, before and after divorce, before and after relocation, before and after multiple sclerosis (MS). Those chapters transitioned from before to after in slow increments, overlapping with other chapters in fairly haphazard fashion.

Before and After Cancer, however, was like a bolt of lightening. Bam! The dividing line, at least the emotional dividing line, is crystal clear. Life was that way, now it's this way, and there's no going back.

On that chilly October night, I wanted nothing more than to crawl into bed and fade into slumber. As I lazily undressed, my left hand brushed over the top of my right breast and landed on a rather large lump. Oh, crap.

I was positive the lump had not been there very long. I would have felt it. I would have known. Certainly, my husband would have found it. Can these things just spring up overnight or had I been completely oblivious? Was I like those women who don't realize they're pregnant until they go into labor? I ran my fingers all around my right breast and the surrounding area, then did the same on the left side. I found nothing else of concern.

Not being the worrying kind, I didn't jump right to a worst-case scenario. I knew the lump was probably the result of a harmless cyst or blocked ducts or some other medical thing I'd never even heard of. Its sheer size and sudden appearance made infection a distinct possibility. It could be any number of things and I knew that cancer was not the most likely scenario.

The soft clacking sounds of fingers on a keyboard told me that my husband, Jim, was still busy in our home office across the hall from the bedroom. He'd be joining me in bed soon, so I took the easy way out, brushing thoughts of the lump aside in favor of a good night's sleep. Surely, it would be gone by morning.

I set the timer on the little television and slid between the cool, white sheets, propping myself up against the pillows. I could see both the TV and Jim from that angle. He reached for the desk lamp and turned out the light. Within minutes, he was cuddled beside me, holding me in his arms as I began to fade.

Sleep came easily and when I woke up, the lump didn't

even enter my mind. Seriously. What can I say? I'm not a morning person. It was a workday, so I headed straight for the shower, still half asleep. The hot water felt good as it hit my face and loosened the tight muscles of my neck. I grabbed the soap and washed my face, then moved down my body, where I rediscovered the ominous Thing That Would Not Be Ignored.

Left to my own devices, I would most likely have waited a few days before reaching out to a doctor. Having MS, it would be an understatement to say I'd had my fill of doctors, and my high-deductible, very expensive individual health insurance policy ensured that I did my best to avoid them whenever possible. Sad, but true.

Jim and I were married shortly after I was diagnosed with MS. He supported me in every way, even rearranging his career to make life more manageable. If he knew about this lump he'd want immediate action, of that there was no question, and I owed it to him. When it comes to my health the man doesn't like to kid around. The wait and see approach was not an option.

Still, I remained silent about the lump and drove across town to my part-time job at a funeral home, where I worked as a correspondence secretary. From there, I called our long-time primary care physician and secured an appointment for Monday. When I broached the subject with Jim, I wanted to show him that I was taking action rather than dismissing it, as I'd dismissed some MS-related concerns in the past.

My gut instincts nagged away at me as I tried to concentrate on work. It would have been so much easier if I could have visited the doctor on my own, in secret, before mentioning it to Jim, but I quickly decided against that plan. It wasn't – and isn't – how our relationship works.

I emerged from my little cubbyhole of an office just as a group of mourners exited the funeral home chapel. I buttoned my blazer, put my head down, and slipped out the side door as quietly as possible. I wanted to get out of the parking lot before the funeral procession began to snake around the building, locking me in place for the duration.

The drive home took only 10 minutes, barely long enough to rehearse how I would approach the subject with Jim. I pictured him sitting at his desk, a target yet unaware of the missile that had been released from its silo.

We met in our kitchen for lunch, leftover salad from last night for me, Italian sausage and peppers for him. Jim enjoyed his lunch while standing at the kitchen sink, calmly looking out at the birds that populated the pine trees lining our yard.

I ate at the table, my foot jiggling as I stared at the painting on the wall and wished I could step inside the picturesque Paris street scene.

When we each had our fill, I breathed deeply and then opened the subject in a manner I thought would convey that everything was under control.

"I've got something to tell you...now, don't get all bent out of shape about this, okay?" *Stupid!* Everyone knows that when you tell someone not to get bent out of shape you're about to give him a reason to get bent out of shape.

"I have an appointment with Dr. R on Monday. I have a lump on my breast. I'm sure it's nothing, but I'm going to get it checked out."

That's when I caught That Look in his eyes. It was an all too familiar mixture of love, concern, and protectiveness that I'd seen so many times before, the look that pierced my heart, the look I hoped never to see again, but there it was. I hated provoking That Look more than I hated the lump.

"Let me see."

I fumbled with the top two buttons of my shirt and led his hand to the lump. It was high on my breast and quite prominent, disturbingly easy to locate. His face froze as his fingers transmitted the troubling new information to his brain.

"Call the doctor back right now. We're going in today," he said in his most serious tone. It wasn't a request.

Guess I didn't convey that "everything's under control" feeling, after all. Knowing better than to argue the point, I made the call, sheepishly telling the receptionist that my husband insisted I see the doctor right away. She managed to squeeze us in, but I wondered what she thought of us.

Here we go again. Most of us who have MS live every single day with that waiting-for-the-other-shoe-to-drop-feeling. Sometimes that other shoe turns out to be a giant, muddy combat boot.

Even though I believed it would ultimately prove to be a false alarm, the irony of the situation was not lost on me. The timing was straight out of a soap opera script.

I was diagnosed with relapsing/remitting MS in 2004. Since then, I had three or four debilitating exacerbations every year, each lasting weeks or months, and seriously affecting every aspect of my life, including my ability to drive and work.

The last major sucker punch occurred in the spring of 2010. Then...nothing. The frequent relapses that plagued me for years disappeared for reasons unknown, and I was enjoying an unprecedented run of vibrant health, thanking the universe and proclaiming this good news to all who would listen. My cane, my handicapped parking placard, and other MS-related helpmates fell into a state of disuse, and I was taking full advantage of the situation.

Sure, I knew the other shoe would eventually drop. I just figured it would be in the form of another MS attack.

Over the summer, I even managed to dance, joining the conga line at my nephew's wedding and romping around with my little nieces, reveling in my role as the goofy aunt from out of town.

I'd finally completed the manuscript for my book, *No More Secs!* Jim and I had been watching the publishing landscape change with the emergence of e-books and self-publishing platforms and decided to publish the book ourselves. Jim was set to begin work on the cover design and coding the book for the electronic version.

My freelance writing portfolio was growing and I was accepted, on the second try, into the American Society of Journalists and Authors. I was feeling very optimistic about writing and my career in general.

On October second, I celebrated my 51st birthday in the best health I'd enjoyed in years. MS was granting sweet relief at last, and I wasn't wasting a moment. I was a full six months into my state-of-remission euphoria.

October is also Breast Cancer Awareness Month. Talk about timing. I was doing my small part by writing and sharing important health information about the disease that had never touched me personally.

No one in my family had ever had breast cancer and I was not aware of any blood relatives who had cancer of any kind. I knew that wasn't a guarantee, of course. I also knew that having MS was no protection against developing additional health problems. Yet I figured I'd have more time, somehow. Figured I'd get a few more good months or maybe even years to feel healthy. Boy, did I figure wrong.

So, I'm glad I danced. I'm glad I giggled and sang and celebrated and appreciated, because life was about to take another turn, and I would need to hold on to those precious moments.

CHAPTER 2

Catch That Look

We entered the examining room at 3:00 p.m. sharp. My breast lump was about to be examined by a doctor for the first time, and I had a very clear idea of how it would go. He would perform a breast exam, tell me it's probably nothing, and write an order for a mammogram, which I was due to have anyway. The lump would be gone by the time I had the mammogram. Easy as one-two-three.

Jim remained in the room as the doctor examined my breasts. He has a sixth sense about these things, that's for sure. The needle on his internal warning system was inching into the red zone. He wanted to make sure things moved along in a timely fashion, and he didn't want me to face the moment alone. I can sometimes be steamrolled, but Jim has a certain strong presence that makes people pay attention. That's a bonus when things go awry. Please pardon my momentary gush, but it's that wonderful combination of confidence and gentleness that makes me love him so.

Our doctor, a D.O., was a no nonsense kind of guy, and while he was appropriately cautious, he wasn't prone to making something out of nothing. That's why the expression on his face was so telling. I hadn't seen that before, not even with the MS. It was concern, yes, definitely concern. Intense concentration. It was an almost imperceptible side-to-side shake of his head that set off my own alarm bells.

He *didn't* say it was probably nothing. He said it was something that needed a closer look...he said it should not wait. He directed his nurse to schedule a diagnostic mammogram as quickly as possible. My last mammogram was performed just 13 months before, so there would be a good comparison.

Despite Jim's anxiety and Dr. R's concern, I was still predicting it would turn out to be nothing. Just another health scare in a long line of health scares. Just another reason for me to get on my soapbox about time-consuming and overly expensive medical tests. Just one more aggravation I'd have to get through.

The receptionist handed me a receipt listing the reason for my visit as "breast lump," causing me to feel slightly sick to my stomach. Somebody somewhere was going type those words into a computer system, where they'd end up on my insurance records. The last thing I needed was another red mark against my name. I felt like a criminal creeping up on the "three strikes and you're out" law. That fear is something that people with employer-based group health insurance don't always understand. There's a little thing called the health insurance death spiral, and I'm pretty sure my plan was gasping for breath.

For the next several days, we kept to our normal routine, but that doesn't mean we had our heads buried in the sand. Without dwelling on cancer, we spoke about the possibilities and agreed, in theory anyway, not to "go there" without reason.

We told no one of our situation. We live in Virginia, while our families, including adult children, are scattered from Rhode Island to Illinois and from New Jersey to New Orleans, so keeping our troubles to ourselves was no great hardship.

Jim is a web developer and he works from our home office. At the time, I worked mornings at the funeral home and as a freelance writer in the afternoons. This precarious balancing act came together as a direct result of my MS and its relentless relapses. We took great leaps of faith to stake out new careers that would enable us to work around my on-again, off-again disabilities.

I was just beginning to toy with the idea of dropping the funeral home job to concentrate on writing full time.

The day before my scheduled mammogram, one of my editors suggested another in a series of articles referencing breast cancer awareness month. I'd never been quite so aware before. In a matter of days I'd become hyper aware, as the line between writing about it and the potential for living it began to blur. I could only hope that after the mammogram on Wednesday, I would be able to chalk it all up to a temporary scare, just a little blip on the line of my life.

We've all heard stories about women who were scared by a false positive test or who worried themselves sick over a lump only to find out it was nothing. Some of them express anger over it. I wanted to be one of those women – not the angry part, the finding out it was nothing part. I decided that if it turned out to be nothing, I'd bypass anger and go straight to gratefulness.

Some women find mammograms painful, but they never really bothered me. After changing into the required upper body gown, I was ushered into the mammogram room and asked to point out the lump. I suddenly became preoccupied with concern about the lump getting squashed in the unforgiving apparatus. I wondered if that could actually happen and what it might mean. For that matter, what if there was an earthquake while my breast was prisoner of the equipment? My mind does take some fanciful leaps.

The lump was so high on my breast that I couldn't imagine how they would even manage to squeeze it in. Ah, those mammograms, they do an excellent job of squeezing, and as far as I could tell, the procedure was routine for the technician.

It was only 8:00 a.m. and I couldn't help glancing at my

watch, still hoping to show up for work on time. My brain continued to classify the situation as a sidebar to my life rather than as part of the main story.

The next stop was another small waiting room where I sat in my lovely gown to await an unseen doctor's opinion. Another woman, also still gowned, was playing the part of Chatty Cathy. She rambled on and on about horses and how she wanted to own her own ranch someday. She looked at me as she spoke, absentmindedly turning the pages of the magazine in her lap, though she wasn't reading it.

She did spin a nice little story, which forced me to focus on her instead of on me. I didn't realize it then, but in retrospect, I suspect she launched into that tale to take her own mind off something she didn't want to think about. I remember her from time to time, and wonder what kind of news she received that day. I hope she is well.

Before too long, a nurse informed me that the doctor wanted to get a better look at my breast by using ultrasound. She gave no hint of urgency as she inquired about my schedule.

Schedule. Work. Routine. It took me about half a second to dismiss my completely irrelevant schedule, as the lump in my breast moved to the very top of my "to do" list. That lump was beginning to get inside my head. We had to resolve it and the quicker the better. It took six months for the MS diagnosis and I did not want to relive that kind of medical limbo, especially when I was feeling so healthy.

"My schedule is clear. I can do it now."

"Okay then, have a seat and I'll be back in a little while."

After phoning the office to report that I'd be late, I called Jim and filled him in.

Stephanie. That was the name of the young, pleasant technician who performed the ultrasound. She took her time and was very thorough, chatting animatedly while expertly maneuvering the wand and capturing image after image on the screen. So many images. It was obvious she took her job seriously, but she remained mindful of the human being involved.

Stephanie was working with an even younger trainee who was carefully observing her mentor. It was when Stephanie turned the wand over to her that I caught it. I saw them exchange That Look, instantly taking me back a few years to when a neurologist exchanged the same type of look with Jim. You know the one I mean – the one where something bad or strange happens and no one wants to vocalize it in your presence. For some reason, they think you won't understand, like when you spell out words in front of your toddler. *"We are not getting a d-o-g."*

As I caught the silent signal meant for her trainee, I internalized the probability that this thing was far from over. Diagnosis or not, right then and there I made an emotional transition, allowing for an infinite array of possibilities and potential outcomes. It's amazing, and a little disconcerting, how calm one can be at such a moment. I was an old pro at compartmentalizing my feelings. It was like my internal filing cabinet had a new folder labeled "breast cancer" among the many other folders of my life, to be opened or filed away as needed.

The team finished their work and I was sent back to the waiting room while the doctor I still had not met reviewed the results. I was beginning to feel as though I'd never make it out of there.

A half hour or so later, I was ushered into the diagnostic radiology department. I followed a nurse to a small, cluttered office where I was introduced, at last, to the mysterious Dr. H, who had been following my tests all morning. It was like pulling back the curtain to come face-to-face with the Wizard of Oz; only this guy was for real.

He offered me a seat and I could see my current mammogram results up on a lighted screen alongside the one from last year. It was a visual confirmation that all was not well. Even a layperson like me could see the obvious changes.

I watched, somewhat detached from my physical self, as he directed my attention to the screen. In his best "It's not good news but I don't want to scare you" voice, the kindly Dr. H informed me that in addition to the large mass I discovered at the 12 o'clock position on my breast, there was another, smaller mass at the 10 o'clock position. Ah, the old one-two punch. I hadn't expected that. What was happening to me?

By the appearance of the mammogram and the ultrasound, he was almost certain we were not dealing with cysts or blocked ducts or any type of infection. He was friendly and empathetic, speaking in a soft, calm voice, but something in his manner implied that he knew more than he was at liberty to say at the moment.

Cancer! The elephant in the room, the *Big C*, whose name remained unspoken, even as his ghostly presence filled the room and engulfed my senses.

Dr. H wanted to biopsy both tumors and asked if I could return the next day. Although I appreciated the fast track, it didn't bode well.

The purpose of the biopsy, he explained, was to obtain tissue samples that would determine if the tumors were malignant or not. Malignant. Another way to avoid the word "cancer."

I don't recall asking many questions about the biopsy. That would be out of character, so perhaps I just don't remember the details. In any case, exactly what would happen in the procedure was lost in the shadows. I gathered my jacket and purse and found my way out to the parking lot, where I paused to let reality sink in. A biopsy tomorrow? With MS, it always seemed to take weeks or months for anything at all to happen. Can't walk? We have an opening three months from now. Tomorrow? These people weren't kidding around.

I phoned the funeral home to say that I wouldn't be in after all. I didn't tell them exactly why, just that I'd been delayed at a doctor's appointment. They'd come to expect my

MS-related absences, so it wasn't a big deal. My duties were not crucial to the operation, anyway.

Jim. I had to go home to tell Jim. Why did I have to keep torturing him? Why did I always seem to be on the verge of disaster? He accepted my MS as part of the package that comes with me. He made it our problem, not my problem. He made adjustments without complaint and struck just the right balance of assistance and respect, keeping our relationship on an equal footing. That's why I wished, with all my heart and soul, that there was a way to spare him this news.

The biopsy was scheduled to take place exactly one week after I first discovered the lump and one way or another, that procedure promised to remove all doubt. It would be my final opportunity to hear that I did not have cancer.

After careful consideration, we decided to keep the cone of silence engaged until we received biopsy results. No sense worrying family over what could still could turn out to be nothing. I could imagine myself telling my mother and my daughter about my eventful days after it all turned out to be a false alarm.

As I snuggled beside Jim that night, I pulled the comforter up high and reminded myself that most breast lumps are noncancerous, but have you ever attempted to rein in a racing mind? The more you try to control it, the more out of control it becomes. My mind was hell-bent on searching for clues, as if that could make a difference.

During the previous month or so, my sleep habits had changed. I found myself waking in the wee hours, unable to go back to sleep. I'd also been feeling a bit fatigued, but was sure it was a precursor to an MS relapse. All in all, I was enjoying the freedom of MS remission without a complaint in the world.

Fear suddenly made its first appearance, as I thought about the numerous hard lumps spread all around my abdomen. What if they were not the result of my daily injections as I had assumed, but were something more sinister? It was time to face the fact that something bad was happening within my body, despite how healthy and strong I felt. It was not the most restful of nights.

Stephanie was back for the biopsy and, like a familiar friend, immediately put me at ease. She and Dr. H worked well together as they prepped me for the procedure. Again, I was struck by their caring manner, and felt a rush of appreciation for that precious gift.

I mentioned to the doctor that I had been dismissing lumps on my abdomen as being caused by injectable MS medication and my concern that I was wrong about that. Much to my surprise, he quickly ran the ultrasound over my abdomen and assured me that those lumps were exactly what I thought they were. He didn't want me to worry needlessly. Finally, there was some encouraging news.

The ultrasound would be used to help pinpoint the two masses. I was positioned with my right arm behind my head and tilted over slightly to my left. It put me in mind of a glamour shot, only without the glamour. It's funny, the things you think about at a time like that.

I shivered as Stephanie applied a cold antiseptic all around my breast area. They offered me a warm blanket, but it was my upper body that was cold, and for that there was no immediate remedy. Then, using a needle, Dr. H gave me a local anesthetic. That was a first for me. Needles in the breast. What a thought. It wasn't terribly painful, but it was definitely unpleasant.

The actual biopsy procedure was very uncomfortable and strange, reminding me of the liposuction I observed on a television program. My poor breast! As instructed, I remained perfectly still as the needle repeatedly probed, seeking the spots that would provide the best tissue samples. The loud, unsettling clacking noise of the equipment seemed to be daring me to move.

The neurologist inserted needles, one at a time, into the muscles of each arm, then into each leg, moving them around while electrodes recorded electrical activity. What seemed like a good idea for a medieval torture device was just part of the diagnostic testing doctors use when they suspect MS. Electromyography, EMG, they call it.

I hated every moment of it, this doctor's manner as cold and detached as if I were a practice mannequin. His only words, spoken in a stern tone, "Don't move."

The larger tumor was easy to get to, but the smaller one was situated more deeply and was difficult to reach, lengthening my discomfort.

I wondered what Jim would think if he could see what was happening to me, that someone was repeatedly shoving a big needle inside my breast and that I was letting him do it. I was grateful that he was out in the waiting room and not allowed to witness the event.

Dr. H and Stephanie seemed to share telepathic messages. They likely already knew that I had cancer, but were still in no position to confirm. Whether they were aware of it or not, I'm not certain, but what they couldn't say in words was conveyed in their manner and in their actions.

After a biopsy, a small metal clip is usually placed in the breast to mark the site for future mammograms. I didn't like the thought of it when Dr. H explained it, but it was not good news when he said I'd had a rough enough morning and he was "letting me off the hook." He said it kindly, with a warm smile, his hand placed gently on my left shoulder, but it was not difficult to decipher the message. Marking the site for future mammograms was not necessary because that particular breast, or at least those parts of it, would not be around very long. Why was I not panicking, or at least crying?

I give Dr. H a lot of credit. His time with the people who come under his care is brief, yet he manages to establish a human connection. It can't be easy.

I wonder if doctors, nurses, and medical technicians realize the power they possess, and how profoundly their demeanor can change everything for the people in their care. They used to call it bedside manner. I call it being human. I will be forever grateful to those medical professionals who understand and practice that. I would never see Dr. H or Stephanie again, but would always remember their professionalism and kindness. As long as you've got to go through something like that, it helps to go through it with good people.

I was disappointed, however, to find that we had to wait until an appointment set a full five days later to receive the results. Things had been happening so quickly that suddenly five days seemed like an eternity. How would we possibly think about anything else?

I rejoined Jim in the outer waiting room. Despite the dozens of other people present, he seemed very much alone. I smiled as I caught his eye. He smiled back. No matter what, there's that.

For the next few days, thoughts of cancer ran on an endless loop through my brain as I went about my daily life. I've known several women who had breast cancer. In each case, the cancer occurred years before I met them, so I never actually had to deal with breast cancer up close. I had zero life experience to tell me how to deal with it. Tuesday could not come soon enough.

Over the weekend, Jim and I attended a friend's birthday party at a local lodge. I'll never forget the feeling of sitting there amidst the laughter and music and food, present in body but only partially present in spirit.

Our friends complimented me on my physical agility, remarking how wonderful it was that I didn't need my cane and how healthy I looked. "Thanks. I feel great!" They had no idea.

Underneath my soft black sweater, hidden from view but

not from mind, dark bruises marked the spots where I'd been biopsied. Despite a festive atmosphere, I could not forget the fact that I was playing host to two sinister lumps in my breast. Lumps made from cells that were dividing and invading and conquering on their quest to take over my body piece by piece, while I sat, smiling and laughing as though it didn't matter.

I wasn't being fake. I had simply compartmentalized my emotions, refusing to allow them to roam freely in public, especially at a friend's birthday party. The file cabinet of my life could keep the cancer folder locked up tightly for a little while longer. There would be plenty of time to open it later.

Jim was similarly preoccupied, but we kept our concerns well hidden behind faces that apparently betrayed nothing. As the celebration continued around us and with us, our eyes had occasion to meet, our unspoken thoughts finding their target.

Love. It's what makes life on this crazy planet worth living.

CHAPTER 3

Head Scarves and Pink Ribbons, Oh My!

Our beautiful backyard had plenty of lush vegetation, pleasing to the eye and to the soul, but in need of constant tending. While Jim was no fan of working out in the heat and humidity, he did enjoy the solitude of hanging out with nature for a few hours each weekend. Unless, of course, his back chose to rebel. When that happened, the pain could last for days, or even weeks.

With one seemingly insignificant reach with a rake, Jim's Sunday commune with nature came to an abrupt halt. When he and his aching back made it into the house, perspiration flowing from under his hat, the pain was evident. Later, his misery was compounded when he accidentally shattered a drinking glass and cut his hand. What a day.

My Monday morning rush to arrive at work on time was complicated by the fact that my car refused to start. As I turned the ignition key, I heard nothing but that sickening sound of silence that every car owner dreads.

Even though it was late October, there was a bee buzzing around my car and making a genuine pest of itself. It was freaking me out in a big way. Do I need a bee sting, too? Can't we catch a break? Jim, bad back and all, had to drive me to work, albeit late again. Things were not running smoothly.

It is human nature, I suppose, to seek signs or to assign meaning to that which has no meaning. Without a superstitious bone in my body, I nevertheless attempted to convince myself that this string of bad luck was a good sign. Yeah, that's it. There *couldn't* be more bad news coming our way, could there? Good news about the lump would even things out nicely and we'd have ourselves a good laugh over the whole thing.

Ah, but the little voice inside my head knew better. The lump in my breast had no relationship with Jim's bad back, a broken glass, a run-in with a bee, or my car's failing engine. The lump in my breast would be what it would be, regardless of other events in our lives. With only one more day to go to get the results of the biopsy, we would know the truth soon enough.

Jim retrieved me from work at 1:00 p.m. and after lunch, I settled in at the kitchen table with my laptop, eager to write my way out of my own head.

At 4:00 p.m., the sound of a ringing telephone interrupted by thoughts. The caller I.D. displayed our primary care doctor's name and I instantly knew we were about to step into Cancer Territory. Prior experience told me that Dr. R does not personally make phone calls to patients unless it is very serious business indeed. He had never called our home before.

What was previously a blurry line between alternate futures was about to sharpen, and I knew it was time to cross that line. All would be changed, as I officially transitioned from "I haven't felt this good in years" to the cancer ward.

I picked up the phone.

"Hello," I answered casually. Somewhere deep down inside, I knew what I was about to hear.

"Is this Ann?" he asked.

"Yes." I dug deep, gathering all available inner strength and putting emotion in check.

"This is Dr. R. I have the biopsy results and I wanted you to hear it from me first." That sentence doesn't usually precede good news. There was a pause as time ceased to exist.

"You have a malignancy and it's very serious. Things are

going to move very quickly now. I would expect you to see a surgeon by the end of the week, and you can count on chemotherapy and maybe radiation. You've got a real tough fight ahead of you."

He said I had cancer. I knew he said I had cancer, but he didn't actually say the word. Not saying it couldn't save me. I don't like to talk around tough subjects by diluting words and robbing them of their impact. I prefer to use the unpleasant words, to feel their raw power so I can face whatever comes from a position of strength.

"So...I have...cancer?"

Hesitation. Then, "Yes."

With my words still hanging in the air, Jim bolted from his office chair and was by my side before the clock could tick another second. We struggled to put the phone in speaker mode, but couldn't make it work, as our fingers fumbled clumsily at the buttons. Heads together, we repositioned the phone between us while the doctor repeated his findings for Jim. He said we were in for a lengthy and difficult process. It was jolting to hear a doctor start out with such a daunting declaration, but it spoke volumes.

Cancer became reality right there in our little kitchen. The very kitchen where Jim proposed to me. The kitchen where our cat, Smokey, took her daily nap in the sunny bay window. The kitchen, with its pale green walls and beat up table that was the heart of our home. The kitchen where we cooked, ate, and laughed every day. The kitchen that would hold a new memory, one that was not pleasant.

Jim put the phone down and we looked at each other in disbelief, finally falling into a long embrace. Time continued to play with our consciousness. Whether we held each other for a minute or for half an hour, I cannot say.

In the movies, this would be the moment where I burst into tears and crumbled to the floor, and it would be completely understandable if I had. But there was no such drama on that most unusual day. Instead, we repeated the doctor's words out loud, making it real and steeling ourselves for something we couldn't possibly understand yet. Why wasn't I freaking out? Why wasn't Jim? Or were we freaking out and just didn't recognize it yet?

I like to tell the story of how I received my MS diagnosis by email. It doesn't get much colder than that. That's why I appreciated the doctor's phone call so much. That kind of news should always be delivered by a human voice.

So, what do you do immediately after hearing you have cancer? Should you take to your bed or run screaming through the streets? Shine the bat signal? I never thought about it before. I suppose if you're in a doctor's office you begin to discuss treatment options. But we weren't in a doctor's office or a hospital. We were home in the middle of a workday.

We sat at the kitchen table. In *No More Secs!*, I wrote that I'm not a "why me?" kind of person. Learning that I had cancer didn't change that, but I'd be lying if I said I didn't experience a brief state of shock that it actually happened, especially while I felt so healthy.

There wasn't much else to say. We still knew little about the cancer. It could be anything from an early stage cancer to a call to start ticking items off my bucket list, but speculating would get us nowhere.

We had to do something! We couldn't just nonchalantly go back to our work. This was BIG! The only thing I could think of to do was to begin making phone calls. Jim went back to his desk, leaving me to the task I felt I must do alone. How he managed to get through the next few hours until dinner, I can't imagine, but there was nothing for him to do until I was ready.

I was not looking forward to telling the family, particularly my children and my mother. How do you tell your family that you have cancer, especially if you live hundreds of miles apart? And when is the right time? We hadn't wanted to worry anyone before the biopsy results, and we still lacked much in the way of information, but there would always be something else to wait for once we were embedded in cancer territory.

At the top of my call list was my daughter. Liz was in her final year of college, and had already decided to stay on for grad school to get her master's degree in behavior analysis. She had her own health issues, those of her boyfriend, and my MS to deal with, and I was about to add to her concerns. As my daughter, she would be more affected by my breast cancer diagnosis than anyone else. Why did I have to give her more to bear?

It was her third birthday party and she was all decked out in her purple Minnie Mouse dress and Minnie Mouse sneakers, her long hair flying in every direction as she ran toward me. With the level of energy only a toddler can summon, she climbed onto my lap and delivered a neck squeeze so tight I momentarily stopped breathing, yet I made no attempt to break her hold. She could hang on forever, as far as I was concerned.

My throat was suddenly as dry as the desert and my eyes began to sting. As I picked up my cell phone, my hand trembled and my stomach weakened. I wanted to sound strong and confident when I told her, so I put the phone down on the wooden table, determined to gather more courage before hitting the speed dial. I stared at the screen on my laptop, wondering how I would do what must be done. Emotions, so neatly held in check through all the preliminaries, were bubbling to the surface, an effect so powerful I felt I could drown.

While I tried to steady my breathing, the phone rang, the usually pleasant-sounding ringtone rattling my nerves. It was Liz, almost as if she felt my angst from halfway across the country. Later, she confessed that she had a strange feeling that compelled her to call me right at that moment. I echoed her happy hello, but she heard it, knew it somehow, so close is our bond.

"What's wrong?"

I tried to answer, but there was a catch in my throat. "Give me a moment," I croaked. Deep breath. More shaking. The back of my throat hurt, but I couldn't fix it. Out with it, then.

"I was just diagnosed with breast cancer." There. My news was out there in the atmosphere, no longer an intangible problem within the confines of our home, but a very real one that would affect other people in our lives. Things were going to change and there was nothing I could do to stop it. I could no longer hold the tears that began a rapid descent down my cheeks. There was no way to cushion the blow.

The brief guttural sound that came through the earpiece tore at my heart. Neither of us is prone to wallowing, so we quickly regained our composure. We weren't about to blubber at each other over the phone, so we had a frank discussion about what we knew so far. In her analytical way, she worked through her questions for which I had few answers, but she offered up her unconditional love. My spirit ached for what I'd just done to her, but I felt an immense sense of relief, too.

"I love you, Mama." I adore the way she calls me "Mama." I could picture her beautiful face, her still long, but now neatly combed hair, and the new worry that would be reflected in her eyes, if only I could see them.

"I love you, too, Sweetie."

That was one of the most difficult phone calls I've ever had to make, but it was only the first of three.

Next, I placed a call to my older son, David.

He needed stitches in his forehead, but he was kicking and fighting the ER doctor. A nurse took baby Elizabeth from my arms so I could hold David's legs still long enough for the doctor to get the stitches in. A moment later, he was suddenly still and oh, so serious. In a loud and accusatory tone he yelled,

24

"What's she doing with my sister?" The nurse stopped in her tracks.

"She's just going to hold her for us until the doctor can finish, so be still, okay, Honey?"

"Okay," he said sternly, if a three year old can be stern. Concern for his sister was all it took to take him outside of himself. Suddenly, there was something more important than the gash in his forehead. He eyed that nurse with unveiled suspicion, but at least the doctor was able to do his work. We were out of there in short order.

No answer. On to younger son, Tommy. As much as I enjoyed speaking with each of them, I wanted this particular string of phone calls to end as quickly as possible.

We sat at the kitchen counter together, little Tommy and I, each with a bowl of chicken noodle soup and some crackers. We were watching "Gullah Gullah Island" as we enjoyed our meal. It was our time, weekday mornings when David and Liz were already in school, and before the bus would arrive to take him off to his afternoon kindergarten class.

"Let's have a chitchat," I'd prompt when the show ended.

"Okay, you be Chit and I'll be Chat," he'd say. And so it went. Conversation is so easy at that age.

He didn't answer, either. As calmly as I could, I left voice mail messages explaining that it was very important they call me back, regardless of time.

I needed to tell them before we could tell anyone else. This was not something I wanted them to learn via the grapevine.

Before the end of the day, they each returned my call, having detected a completely unfamiliar tone in my voice.

It was a dreadful chore, telling my children. It was my job to be there for them, the net under their high wire act, but things weren't working out that way. Instead, they were the ones who offered reassurance and support. Their warmth and strength of character soothed my aching heart.

Not only do I live far from my children, I live far from my mother, too. How do you call your elderly mother who lives alone and tell her you have cancer? It was difficult enough to tell her about the MS back in 2004. This was going to be many times worse. I couldn't stand the thought of her being alone when she heard that her daughter had cancer. It would be much better if someone could tell her in person, I reasoned. So, I hatched a plan.

I phoned my eldest brother, taking him a bit by surprise when I said, "I'm calling because I need my big brother."

Growing up, siblings are just as likely to annoy the hell out of each other as they are to offer comfort after a bad day. Things change in dramatic ways as you mature and forge separate lives. For us, no matter how far apart we've lived or how seldom we've managed to get together, there is an unspoken bond between us, a deep connection that cannot be broken.

"What do you need?" There was an abundance of caution in his voice. I had no doubt he would do just about anything for me, but he was aware that I don't make a habit out of asking for help. He knew, instinctively, that something had to be terribly, terribly wrong, and he was ready to respond.

I got right down to it. "I was just diagnosed with breast cancer." He was understandably shocked, but shifted with ease into big brother mode. He'd had his own share of tough times in life and wanted to help in any way he could. He listened carefully as I explained what we knew so far, and how I wanted him to go tell Mom personally. I asked him to tell my sister as well. He could get them together and tell them both at once. Then they could call me when they were ready to talk.

After some discussion, we agreed that I would call him again the next day, after my scheduled appointment at the hospital. Perhaps then I'd have more details to offer. In the meantime, he would break the news to my grown nieces and nephew, one of whom called me within minutes. I felt a sense of relief and peace, knowing that my brother was taking charge on the home front.

With that heavy weight off my shoulders for the moment, I turned to dinner preparation. As was my habit, I cranked up the music and sang, moving with the rhythm while I cooked. Just another ordinary day in which extraordinary things took place.

After dinner, we went outside to give my ornery Grand Am a jump-start so it would be ready for my morning commute. All in all, it was not an unproductive day. As evening rolled in, we settled in on the sofa to watch television. That sofa was our comfort zone at the end of each day, the place where we wound things up and enjoyed the simple pleasure of being together.

We considered making popcorn, which is our favorite evening snack, but I had a sudden, very unusual craving. "I wish we had some ice cream."

After a few moments of discussion about the wisdom of junk food at 9:00 p.m., or the wisdom of junk food at all when you've just been told you have cancer, we decided that if you can't go out for ice cream on the day you learn you have cancer, when can you? Nobody declared me dead. If, as the doctor said, we were in for a tough fight, why not indulge ourselves a bit?

We grabbed our jackets and headed for the car. A couple of scoops did the job nicely.

We arrived at the busy hospital at the scheduled time on Tuesday afternoon to discuss the biopsy results. The receptionist checked the schedule, looked down at her shoes, and mumbled something about needing a nurse to come get us. Obviously, hospital staff had a procedure to follow and they were going through the formal motions required.

If we *had* been unaware, the nurse with the prominent American Cancer Society (ACS) badge on her chest would have been the first tip-off. What an awful moment that would have been had I not already known. I was more grateful than ever that my doctor chose to call and tell me himself. Finding out this way would have been a cruel awakening. The hospital could use some sensitivity training on that point.

The ACS nurse seated us in a cramped, oh, so bland private room and mumbled something about finding "a" doctor to speak with us. I don't know why, but I had assumed we would be speaking with Dr. H, and I was thrown by the awkwardness of this meeting. She needed an M.D. to make it all official, but it apparently didn't matter who or how. I'm not blaming the nurse or the ACS, but the process that was supposed to help patients through a difficult meeting was poorly executed.

"A" doctor quickly introduced himself, but both Jim and I forgot his name the instant he said it, so surreal was the moment. He gave the paperwork a cursory glance. His delivery was rushed and without feeling. "Well, you've got a malignancy and it's not good. The smaller tumor is not cancerous, but the larger one is. The first thing you need to do is choose a surgeon," he said, indicating a list of surgeons taped to the dull gray wall.

So matter-of-fact was he about cancer. *About my cancer. My life!* Not a trace of caring or concern. It was almost as if he was telling me I had a scraped knee and needed a bandage, so what color did I want?

From "you have cancer" to "pick a surgeon." Surely, we would need more details. Wasn't that why we were here?

The list of surgeons included headshots and looked more like the FBI's Ten Most Wanted list than a list of potential lifesavers. To our questions about the qualifications and reputations of the surgeons, he replied that it really didn't matter which one we chose because "they're all good."

We inquired about urgency and he replied that speed is not as important as choosing the right doctor. Hmmm…is it just me or is that a peculiar circle of logic?

This particular doctor's job was to officially deliver medical news to a patient he never met before and would never see again. Clearly, that job was complete, and he left us with the nurse. He didn't offer any further information, nor did he give us the opportunity to ask questions. I don't think he could have identified me in a lineup five minutes later. Then again, I couldn't identify him, either. There was a white coat, but it was occupied by a dispassionate life form that made no lasting impression.

We had some terrible experiences with health care in the previous few years. So much so, that I had begun to back away from doctors, making appointments only when absolutely necessary. This was a matter of self-preservation, a move meant to alleviate the stress of living with MS, as well as the enormous expense of it all.

"A" doctor was probably oblivious to the fact that he was setting such a negative tone and ratcheting up our stress level. Either that, or he truly didn't give a damn. It was actually painful to imagine that more of the same awaited us. I made a silent vow not to stand for any doctor who didn't see me as a fellow human.

The nurse seemed somewhat embarrassed by the doctor's performance, but forged ahead purposefully, meeting our eyes and doing her best to make up for his carelessness. She introduced herself again, and said she would be coordinating things and working with the various doctors on our behalf. It sickened me a bit, to think that this would be so complicated that I'd need a coordinator. She told us that she was a cancer survivor herself, plus she had three other patients who also have the double whammy of MS and breast cancer. She was attempting to form a bond.

Reviewing the biopsy report, she put her hand to her forehead and rubbed it slowly, thoughtfully, as if unsure of what to say or how to say it. "You don't see triple-negative very often..." her voice trailed off. It was the first time we heard the phrase "triple-negative," but without further explanation, the significance of that term was lost on us for the time being.

Jim wasn't about to settle for that "they're all good" nonsense and began asking questions of the nurse. It was like trying to snatch a bone from a pit bull's jaws. In typical "I can't tell you what I really think" fashion, she went out of her way not to recommend anyone in particular.

When we finally chose a surgeon, it turned out he couldn't see us for three months. When I think back, I'm appalled that neither the doctor nor the nurse conveyed any sense of urgency, knowing that I had triple-negative breast cancer. Fortunately, the prospect of waiting three months – no matter what kind of cancer I had – was completely unacceptable to us.

We went through the list again. Our second fairly random choice, Dr. M, had some time set aside each day for new and urgent cases, and could see us in just a few days. All we knew of her was where she went to medical school, where she interned, and that she had a good reputation in town. It was a place to start, anyway.

The nurse explained that I would probably need a lumpectomy and a check of my lymph nodes to see if the cancer had spread. Only then could it be "staged." Then we would have a clearer picture of what we faced. That's when we would be able to formulate the specifics of my treatment plan.

Jim made it clear to her that he was willing to do anything and take me anywhere for the best treatment. He's a man of action and he was becoming frustrated with the uselessness of this meeting. She promised to help us with anything we night need in the future. She seemed sincere and I'm sure we would have contacted her if we found the need. In reality, we would never call upon her again. We didn't need or want a coordinator.

The appointment with our prospective surgeon was scheduled for that Friday, and we were fairly anxious. We didn't want any delay. We didn't expect to learn much more then, but hoped to come away with a surgery date, at the very least. I wanted to get the cancer out of my body as quickly as possible.

We departed the hospital knowing little more than when we went in, but we were armed with a copy of the biopsy report. We could begin research on our own to find out what we were up against.

The report gave us some important information about the cancerous tumor, making it more real...and a lot more intimidating. The tumor was listed as "infiltrating moderate-poorly differentiated ductal carcinoma." That meant the cancer cells bore little resemblance to normal breast cells. It was invasive and cancer had spread from where it started into surrounding breast tissue, and potentially beyond.

My tumor tested negative for progesterone receptors, negative for estrogen receptors, and HER-2 negative. That's how triple-negative breast cancer gets its name.

All these new words entering our vocabulary, and so very much to learn on our own.

Another round of phone calls and we were fairly exhausted with the process. I spoke to my brother, who had the unfortunate task of telling my mother and sister, and then I spoke to each of them. I had visions of my brother in action from afar, rallying family in support. I definitely called on the right guy.

At work the next morning, I filled my boss in on my health status, since I'd be taking time off work for surgery soon. I also sent emails to some of my regular writing clients, letting them know that there could be lapses in communication, but I would remain on the job. And so began the watched pot stage, when people started to look at me as if waiting for water to boil.

Wouldn't you know it? On Friday morning, my car failed to start again. Jim had to drive me to work, and then pick me up so we could head over to the surgeon's office. Life doesn't cut you any slack for having MS or cancer.

After our experience with "a" doctor the other day, Dr. M was a much-appreciated breath of fresh air. Her front office staff and her nurse were all kindness and light, easing our tensions at the outset.

We entered the inner office and, in a first for us, Dr. M greeted us each with a genuine hug and a sincere smile.

Again, Jim was present as she performed a physical exam. After I was dressed and seated next to Jim, she placed the biopsy report in front of us and wrote the words, "triple-negative," pointing at them as she spoke.

She explained that because triple-negative breast cancer is negative for hormone receptors, we had fewer treatment options. Some of the more recent therapies, like tamoxifen, were rendered useless to me. She stressed that surgery and chemotherapy were excellent weapons against triple-negative breast cancer.

She used the phrase "your cancer" multiple times, as if to make sure we would soak that in. Doctors who care take the time to assess a patient's state of mind before plunging head-long into talk of removing body parts. Dr. M is one of those. Jim, sensing that she was leading us somewhere in particular, decided to clear the way for her.

"You can tell us straight out. We've done some research. We get how serious this is – and we want this thing out. We'll do whatever it takes and go wherever we have to, to make sure she lives through this. You don't have to cushion anything for us."

Dr. M smiled, satisfied that she could continue with her deliberate, honest assessment. She didn't whitewash the situation, but neither was she the least bit discouraging. She was telling us that this cancer – my cancer – was not a slow-growing cancer for which we could take a wait and see approach. She was telling us that we needed to be as aggressive and fast moving as it was.

Lumpectomy, she said, was not an option. That was the headline. That's what she needed to get across. She knew I'd be expecting a lumpectomy.

The large and aggressive cancerous tumor, its location, the presence of the second tumor, and the relative size of my breast all factored into her recommendation for a mastectomy.

The size of the tumor indicated a minimum of stage two, possibly three, she told us.

She explained how the large tumor appeared dangerously close to penetrating the chest wall, a very serious situation, so an MRI of the chest would be necessary before attempting surgery. None of us broached the topic of what it would mean for me if the cancer had already entered a lung. One thing at a time.

Despite our shock, a tentative surgery date of November 10 was put on the calendar. I was going to lose my breast. I hadn't expected that, at least not so soon. Hadn't I just found the lump? And no lumpectomy? How could I already be at stage three? There was a sense of urgency in the air.

Dr. M strongly suggested that we not concern ourselves with preparing for reconstructive surgery at this time, if ever. She didn't want anything to get in the way of a clear view of my breast area and chest wall for the foreseeable future. I was beginning to get the picture. I was not fighting to save my breasts. I was already fighting for my life.

The look of confidence and concern on her face made me trust her. We already knew that her husband was a surgeon who specialized in breast reconstruction, so for her not to recommend reconstruction was quite telling.

She appreciated our queries and our desire to move quickly. Life over breast was agreed upon by all. Jim and I were already way beyond concerning ourselves with the cosmetics of it all, anyway.

Though undeniably sobered by the sequence of her recommendations, a sense of cool, calm purpose fell over us.

"You're already a survivor," Dr. M pointed out. "From the moment you were diagnosed, as long as you are alive, you are a survivor."

A survivor. As long as I am alive. Visions of eyebrow-less women wearing head scarves and pink ribbons danced into my consciousness. Apparently, I was one of them now, but I didn't feel like one of them. Then again, who does? Me? A survivor? Somehow, I didn't feel I deserved the label. It didn't take long to go from finding a suspicious lump to being called a survivor. Shouldn't you have to go through something big to call yourself a survivor? If not, aren't we all survivors just for making it through another day?

Next thing you know, someone's going to say I died after a "courageous battle" with cancer, I thought. They never say it was a "cowardly retreat," or "she was scared out of her mind." The battle part seemed completely appropriate, but that whole courageous thing was yet to be determined.

I was scheduled for a chest MRI on Monday morning, and could expect results on the following day.

After asking about my work situation, she said that in the months to come, I might have difficulty keeping up. Things felt more serious by the minute.

Dr. M assured us she would forward all this information to a highly recommended oncologist who would meet with us several weeks after surgery. He would explain the post surgery options of chemotherapy and radiation.

After giving us a breast cancer guidebook on which she scrawled her home phone number, she ended our session with another round of hugs. Yes, you read that right. She gave us her home phone number. We would never use it, but simply having it was of great comfort. Beyond her surgical scalpel and prescription pad, this doctor is a true healer, and I'll be forever grateful.

From Dr. M to the nurse to the woman who handled our paperwork, we were pleasantly surprised by the very real connection we felt with this group. Our cancer team was coming together, aiming for a win. We knew we were in good hands.

So much about triple-negative breast cancer remained unsaid, but we continued our research. We learned that this type of breast cancer tends to be more aggressive than other types, and is more likely to spread beyond the breast and recur after treatment, especially in the first five years. That's why five-year survival rates tend to be lower. After that time, it averages out with other types of breast cancer. It would be a formidable opponent.

Calling my family with updates was becoming a matter of routine. These details were difficult to share, especially with my children, but I didn't want to blindside anyone by filtering out the hard truth. If we must do this thing, we would not be pulling our punches.

CHAPTER 4

The Waiting Days

We were occupying that space between knowing life was about to change in a profound way and life actually changing. This new territory was uncharted, at least by us. I felt healthy and strong in spite of it all, adding to the surreal atmosphere that was our world.

Our normal routine remained intact, but there was an underlying sense of restlessness. We kept our attention on practical matters.

At work, the confines of my small office were becoming intolerable, the hours until 1:00 p.m. ticking off at a snail's pace. It felt wrong, somehow, to spend half a day without seeing the sun or the sky. Jim was concentrating on keeping ahead of his own work. At least it appeared that he was concentrating. It is more likely that his mind was as cluttered and unfocused as my own.

By careful design, our home had an uncluttered, peaceful feeling, and we wanted it to stay that way. It's easier on the body and on the spirit. So, chores weren't pushed aside. Laundry. Vacuum. Dust. Tidy.

When a storm is forecast, one stocks up on food. It's a habit formed during the winter snows of my New England upbringing. For whatever reason, having a fully stocked kitchen makes me feel prepared, so we filled up on staples, stocking the cupboards and refrigerator. In the meantime, we still had to eat. Chop the carrots, toss the salad, season the fish. Wash the dishes, wipe the countertops. Routine.

Shouldn't we be doing something important with these days, I wondered? Checking items off a bucket list, perhaps? Making hasty plans to visit the kids? Really, what should a person do at a time like that? We had no game plan. We were both flying by the seat of our pants.

I thought about what else might help get me through the next few weeks and we set off on a shopping trip. I chose some cozy fleece pants, loose cotton tees, and a couple of hoodies that zip up the front for the post-surgery era.

It may seem ridiculous that we would spend these days performing such mundane chores, but it helped me to feel prepared for surgery and recovery, as though I was moving things forward rather than simply waiting for time to tick by. Beyond these things, there was nothing else we could do to get ready, as the possibilities were infinite.

We began to hear from far-off relatives and friends and I truly felt for them. Most didn't quite know what to say, which is completely understandable. The fact that someone reaches out at all is good enough.

Already relationships were beginning to alter their course. We would soon learn that cancer affects relationships in surprising ways. Cancer brings out the best and the worst in people. A few people we thought were friends...weren't. Some people are simply unable to deal with cancer and fade away like so many shadows in the night. No call or acknowledgement of that which has so shaken your world. This is sometimes later explained away as, "I didn't want to bother you..."

Others I barely knew, some complete strangers, reached out from the far corners of the globe to simply say, "How are you?" It's an up close and personal study of human nature, for better or worse.

When you go through a life-altering event such as cancer or MS, it helps to realize that the reactions of others say nothing at all about you. It says something about them. It's about their awkwardness or fear or inability to find the right words, or about their kindness and empathy toward a fellow human being. Cancer, or even the possibility of cancer, forces us to confront the core of who we are and how we relate to others. It reminds us of our finite time on earth, something many of us would prefer to ignore.

If I may impart one bit of wisdom on the subject, it is this: make the call; send the card; stop by and say hello – even if you haven't a clue what to say. To shy away because you feel awkward is a mistake and the longer you wait, the harder it will be to rectify. You will come to regret it.

Prior to my cancer diagnosis, I'm not sure I could have identified my mail carrier in a crowd. I hardly ever caught more than a glimpse of her as she made the rounds of our neighborhood. One day, she left a post card in our mailbox. She wanted me to know that she heard about my cancer through our neighbor and that her mother had been through the same ordeal. She simply wanted to wish me well and let me to know she was thinking of me.

That simple act of kindness was good medicine, indeed. That post card remains one of my most cherished possessions and a perfect example of how a simple gesture from the heart can mean so much.

I knew my cancer would be hard on Liz, but I didn't fully realize her struggle until the day she said, "I wish it was me, instead." Now there's a statement that'll rip a mother's heart right out. Perish the thought. Better the mother than the daughter, without question.

During those days, the waiting days, my thoughts inevitably turned to the future – and the possibility that mine would be shortened. Would I live to see my children marry or have children of their own?

Would I be around to see them achieve their career goals? David, armed with a master's degree, was just beginning his business career. Liz was highly engaged in her field of study, working toward a career helping people with developmental disabilities. Tommy, in the persona of his wrestling alter egos

("The Famous" Justin Reno and Jester Judas Yorick), was wowing the crowds on the independent wrestling circuit. I wanted to be part of it all, to watch as they spread their wings.

Now don't get me wrong – I wasn't giving up by any stretch of the imagination. I had every intention of fighting for all of these things, but I'm also a realist. Jim and I would not pretend that the possibility of death was nonexistent, especially between the two of us. After all, it's hard to dismiss death when you work in a funeral home. It was not a taboo subject for us. We felt free to say anything – and we did.

Death is part of life. Ignoring the possibility of death will not prevent it and addressing it will not hasten its appearance. Death knows no rules about age or fairness or timing. At the funeral home, I saw far too many young people snatched from life before having the chance to live.

As we went about the details of planning for surgery, recovery, and continued treatment, we also considered the worst-case scenario – not in a maudlin or overly fearful way, but for practical purposes. We would hope for and work toward the most favorable outcome and a long life together, while acknowledging the possibility of death. I wanted my affairs in order; I wanted my wishes known; I felt better for having done so.

Our conversations about death did us a world of good. Because there was no pretense that the possibility didn't exist, we were able to get to the real task at hand – living. Jim and I are positive people, and we are nothing if not warriors. We are realistic optimists, and that has always served us well.

I was – and am – a very fortunate woman, to have a husband who could look me in the eyes and tell me that he loves me...me...with MS, and with or without breasts or hair or any other physical changes that may come. He loves me...of that there is no doubt. And I know he feels my love in return.

There was so much for me to ponder in those waiting days, my thoughts taking off on flights of fancy I could not control. At times I would snap out of deep introspection, unable to recall where my thoughts had been just moments before. I read whole pages of books without grasping a word, watched movies without hearing the dialogue or recalling the plot.

All the while, Jim was a man in pain, quietly enduring hellish thoughts I could only imagine.

The questions were bound to surface. Did you keep up with mammograms? Did you smoke? Is there breast cancer in the family? Did you eat your veggies? Yes, no, no, and yes. I suspect that people who ask these questions want evidence to confirm they're doing everything right, but this I could not offer. I was at low risk for breast cancer in general and didn't fit the typical profile of someone at risk for triple-negative breast cancer.

Cancer really makes you think about all the chemicals and products you've been exposed to throughout your lifetime. I had the same thought process when diagnosed with MS. I'll never know exactly why I had this type of cancer and will always worry about my children.

Sunday was Halloween and we ran a few errands, trying to maintain some order in the physical realm while chaos ruled our minds. We also dropped my car off so it could be serviced on Monday. I was feeling increasingly fatigued and my lower legs and feet throbbed. I could only hope that my MS was not about to make an entrance.

After dinner they began to arrive. Ghosts and monsters, sports heroes, and a parade of pink princesses, holding their bags open in anticipation of treats.

With each ring of the doorbell, Smokey ran for cover while Jim and I took turns delivering the expected goods and oohing and ahhing at the little ones' antics. A nice distraction, to be sure, but this Halloween felt different somehow, as if I watched from afar rather than participated. My physical body, with its own resident monster, was present and accounted for, but my mind occupied a thousand universes all at once.

David was all decked out in his black knight costume, complete with plastic sword, and Liz wore a shiny pink mermaid outfit. Picking out the right costume took some time and this was the first Halloween that Liz was able to anticipate the fun of trick-or-treating around the neighborhood.

Wouldn't you know it? David suddenly spiked a fever. After taking the obligatory photo and visiting our neighbors' house, his knighthood came to an abrupt halt. It was pajamas and a cozy blanket for him, and he was so tired he didn't even fuss about it. Fortunately, my dear friend from across the street offered to take Mermaid Liz along with her boys. Good neighbors are a treasure.

I recalled the year it was so frightfully cold in Chicago's northwest suburbs that even the kids wanted to go back home after half a block; and the year that it was raining and so violently windy that my umbrella turned inside out and flew from my cold hands. I remembered the unseasonably warm Halloween when my neighbor and I pushed strollers down the street as the older kids pranced around in their costumes and gathered treats. I thought about how recently those events took place and how fleeting those years were.

Aside from Jim's, it was the faces of the nurses and doctors that appeared and reappeared in my mind's eye. Since I didn't have the visual reactions of my family, these were the faces I connected with. Compassionate faces. Helpful faces. Knowing faces. I was always terrible with names, forgetting most as soon as they are spoken, but I knew those names and those faces and especially those eyes.

Pete was his name and he would perform the MRI of my chest on Monday. Because of recent shoulder problems, I feared I wouldn't be able to relax my arms in the required position, but the cute little pills the doctor gave me did the trick. Actually, it did the trick a little too well.

I was so relaxed that I dozed off during the MRI, but apparently, all went smoothly. As soon as we returned home, I took a nap. Jim woke me up at 11:00 a.m. and I made some soup. Then I fell asleep again until 2:30 p.m. I'm such a lightweight when it comes to medication that I was completely done in.

We planned to go pick up my car at 5:00 p.m., when all the medication would be out of my system, but I never did feel ready to drive. What a crazy day – and we weren't even at the starting gate, yet. We brought out some leftovers for dinner so I wouldn't have to cook, and we enjoyed a light meal.

Jim's daughter and her husband phoned to say they'd be in the area over the weekend and wanted to visit, which just about lit up our world. Family! The timing couldn't be better.

Shortly after that, my brother called to tell me that he, my sister, one of my nieces, my nephew and his wife, and my mother would be driving down from Rhode Island to visit over the same weekend.

It was a rare treat, but I suppose they wanted to feel as though they were doing something, and it would be good for them, too, I realized. They should see me while I still look like me. What a pleasant way to pass the waiting days! My mother doesn't care for travel, so this was a huge deal and I was beside myself with joy. My energy level rose with the anticipation of company.

Tuesday morning was voting day for the mid-term elections, so we began the day at the polls, then went to pick up my newly repaired car so I could go to work.

We met with Dr. M later that afternoon. Sometimes good news is just not worse news and we finally had some "not worse" news. Although there was only a very thin layer of tissue between the tumor and my chest wall, it appeared that it had not penetrated the lung. She couldn't say it with 100 percent certainty until the actual surgery, of course, but she was very encouraged – and encouraging.

I could actually see the muscles of Jim's face relax for the first time in days, and he breathed a visible sigh of relief. Finally, we had some good news to report to family, and I spent all afternoon on the phone.

She also said that my left breast looked absolutely "pristine." What a good word, pristine. After that, I began to refer to my left breast as Pristine, or "Prissy" for short. A little silliness goes a long way.

The next fly in the ointment was the fact that I'd managed to pick up a head cold, and if I couldn't kick it, or if it settled in my chest, surgery would have to be postponed. With pre-operative tests scheduled for Monday afternoon and the mastectomy of my right breast scheduled for Wednesday, that didn't leave me much time to fight it off. The cold would have to go, because I couldn't stand the thought of giving the cancer more time to penetrate that thin wall.

Besides all the concern for my health and my life and all the emotion that goes with that, another issue was nagging away at me. Health insurance. With my premiums increasing annually at a rate of 25-35 percent, my fear was not unfounded. As it was, our monthly health insurance premium was the biggest line item in our budget, beating out our mortgage payment. That high price tag came with a $5,000 deductible each, various co-pays, and a 40 percent co-pay on prescriptions, which didn't count toward the overall deductible. Dental and vision coverage not included. Still, if it would cover the bulk of my cancer treatment, it would make all the difference in the world.

My fears ratcheted up a notch when an envelope from my health insurance carrier landed in my mailbox. It would not be an exaggeration to say that my heart was pounding as I opened the envelope, certain that some new horror was about to befall me. Instead, I read:

> "Health care reform is now law. [...] You are eligible for the following benefits beginning on January 1, 2011: No lifetime dollar limits or maximums."

I closed my eyes and came just short of crying with relief. What it meant at that particular time in my life is difficult to put into words. The new benefit was of no small comfort. Whatever was to come, at least I wouldn't be cut off. One less thing to worry about.

Emotions can change so quickly. By Wednesday evening, I felt a growing, seething anger. I accepted that I had cancer. I accepted that it was a particularly aggressive type. I even accepted that I must lose a breast. What I couldn't accept was the cruel timing of the head cold.

I had to be rid of it before surgery could take place. Time mattered, and any delay could be disastrous. A domino effect could lead to death by cold, I reasoned. Of course, that's an incredible stretch, but it's all part of cancer's mind games.

The cold was messing with my ability to enjoy my last remaining days as a two-breasted woman. A little dramatic, perhaps, but I was overdue for dramatics. The cold was the catalyst that finally freed the emotion from its prison, and the emotion was anger. Was it too much to want to spend a couple of nice days with family before heading off into the great unknown?

We had only a few days left before surgery and its aftermath. Coughing, sneezing, and sniffling were constant reminders of how precious that time was. There was no one to be angry with, of course, so I was forced to push those thoughts aside and concentrate on getting stronger.

God, the universe, nature, or random chance...however human beings came to be, whatever label you want to put on it, life is a gift. Part of that gift is the beauty of the human body, the places it can take us, and the amazing things it can do.

In my younger years, I didn't appreciate this body or see its natural beauty. By the time I hit my mid forties, I had come to fully embrace it, flaws and all, finally seeing it for the work of art it is. I'd kept myself in pretty good shape for a 51-year-old mother of three with MS, but losing a breast wasn't something I took lightly.

It was a rough night. Dreams of my breasts invaded my sleep. I saw myself with two breasts, then with one missing. I love balance and symmetry and felt thoroughly unsettled by the thought of my impending one-sidedness. I tried to stay awake so as not to dream it again, but dreaming was not required. The thoughts pressed on even while I was awake.

I was also pre-mourning the loss of my hair. The things that are generally associated with femininity and female sexuality would be mine no longer.

We are, all of us, more than our physical bodies. My breasts had a mighty good run. I decided I would no longer think in terms of losing a breast, but as saving my life. Balance comes from within and I would retain mine, with or without the usual number of breasts or a full head of hair. This old body of mine is a real trouper.

There's a tee shirt with the slogan, "Yes they're fake. My real ones tried to kill me." That's not how I wanted to look at it. I didn't want to blame my breasts or my own body. I decided the old girl was taking one for the team. She's a heroine, that's what she is.

Nobody *wants* to lose a breast. But when that perfect storm of circumstances blows in and your life is at stake, it's not a hard decision to make. The fact is, femininity is all in your head. Or rather, in your brain. So is your sexuality. If you choose breast reconstruction, prosthetic breasts, or to remain just as you are, you are still you.

The same goes for hair. If you go bald due to chemotherapy, wear a hat or a wig, or never regain your former luscious locks, if you take a good look in the mirror – I mean really look into your own lash-less eyes, you'll see the truth. Your feminine spirit is untouched by physical changes, and that's a mighty powerful feeling. You're all woman.

Jim and I were looking forward to our sixth anniversary in February, still newlyweds in many ways. This wasn't the first physical challenge we faced, and obviously wouldn't be the last. We have yet to meet the foe that can come between us. Even breast cancer would not succeed in that.

I was making my peace with the changes to come. I was mentally prepared to remove the cancerous cells from my body before they could cause more harm.

A 3:00 a.m. coughing jag rescued me from my dreams and jumbled thoughts. Off to the living room sofa I went, sleeping on and off in front of the television, wrapped up in my favorite cozy throw blanket.

When the morning alarm sounded, Jim got up with purpose. "This is your caregiver speaking. There is no way you are going to work today."

In our home, Jim is in charge of breakfast. He whipped up a batch of hot oatmeal. Not the instant kind that comes in an envelope filled with added sugars, mind you, but the good old-fashioned kind that you prepare on the stovetop.

After serving me a bowlful, he sent me back to bed, which turned out to be a great idea. Restful sleep came at last and set things right once again.

If he could have switched places with me, he would have done so in a heartbeat. I'd never seen Jim so...I'm not sure what word to assign it. The man loves me and he loves our life together. He will accept me in any shape I happen to be in, but I'll venture to say he was scared to death.

People tend to underestimate the toll of serious illness on the spouse. Almost all the attention and support is geared toward the one with the illness. In many ways, it is the spouse who could use a little help and understanding.

I hoped he would receive the support he needed throughout the ordeal. He carried a lot of weight on his shoulders, weight I could not help him bear.

It was one of those quiet dinners married people have. Music gently played in the background, accompanied by the clinking of forks and plates, but no conversation. We hadn't had a falling out and neither of us was upset. It's inevitable that two people who are together almost all the time sometimes run out of chatter.

I used to cringe when I saw that couple in a restaurant. Must be horrible, I thought then, but I know better now. When a relationship is good...truly good...you don't need chatter all the time just for the sake of chatter or to fill a perceived void. There is no void. Sometimes words only get in the way of the simple pleasure of being together.

I was looking a bit disheveled after my morning nap. I hadn't had time to fix myself up properly when Liz initiated a Skype video call. Were it not for cancer, I probably would have begged off until I could put myself together. The sudden and monumental shifts caused by cancer made me realize how unimportant some things are. Having a video chat with my daughter easily trumped my less-than-captivating appearance.

My nose ran and I coughed throughout our chat. I'm sure it wasn't a pretty sight, but it felt good to connect face-to-face. When I apologized for my appearance, she replied, "Now *that's* the Mommio I know so well..." One could take that statement a number of ways, but I had to laugh in spite of myself.

On Friday, we cautioned our incoming guests to proceed at their own risk for the weekend. I truly did want to visit with each and every one them, yet didn't want to get anyone sick.

The scale showed a six-pound weight loss in a couple of weeks. I had noticed a slight loss of appetite, but not enough to lose six pounds in such a short time. That couldn't be a good sign. I didn't have many extra pounds to spare. Maybe an active weekend with family would help.

Jim's daughter and her husband drove in from New Jersey and arrived first. We were sitting around the living room, having a wonderful visit, when the Rhode Island contingent showed up. Within a matter of moments, our quiet home was transformed into a full house, alive with conversation and laughter. Cold or no cold, they all wanted to be there and there wasn't a hint of gloom or doom. Our home was so full of life!

I don't get the chance to visit with my family as often as I would like. I moved away shortly after my 22nd birthday. Our relationships have been based on whirlwind visits ever since. I have two brothers who live in Texas, and I see them even less frequently.

We all trooped down to a local Chinese restaurant for dinner. It was a rare occasion, this blending of our families, and there was no reason to bring up cancer. When you don't live near family, you come to place great importance on events that others take for granted. You notice every laugh, every little nuance, and everything that reminds you of where you came from and how you're connected on the tree of life.

Saturday's weather was cool and wet, the skies gray, but spirits remained high. The weekend was probably as cathartic for everyone else as it was for me. It's not that we did a lot. For the most part, we sat around, talking, catching up, and simply enjoying each other's company.

The gang presented me with a gift, my first eReader, thinking it would be a handy thing to have around in the months to come. They were right on the money with that thought. It became my constant companion in waiting rooms and during the long months of chemotherapy and beyond.

It was a slightly different feeling on Sunday, as the family prepared to hit the road. We went out for a hearty breakfast, and then gathered in the parking lot to say our goodbyes. That's when cancer rejoined the party.

With tears in her eyes, my sister said she would take the cancer for me if she could and of that, I had no doubt. Wow. My daughter, my husband, and my sister, all wishing to take the burden. It might not be so impressive if they were just empty words, but I knew in my heart that none of them made the statement lightly. It was, as you might expect, time for tears and heartfelt expressions of love.

The thing is, I wouldn't want any of them to take my cancer, and I'm a lot stronger than any of them could possibly know. Maybe even stronger than I knew at the time.

As they started off on their northbound journey, we stood waving until we could see them no longer. They must have been wondering if they would ever see me that way again, or maybe even if they'd ever see me again at all. I know I was.

With only a few days to go, Jim and I spent the afternoon wrapped in each other's arms. My cold was already easing and we knew I'd be approved for surgery.

Just before bedtime, I felt a wave of sadness, a brief feeling of mourning. Jim was very comforting, assuring me that he loved me for who I am and that will never change. I believed him. His tender touch and his sweet caress swiftly eased my sadness. Nothing in life matters so much as love.

CHAPTER 5

Pristine Stands Alone

On Monday, it was back to work for me. It's funny how something can be so normal and so abnormal at the same time. Trying to carry on with our regular schedule seemed like the right thing to do, especially since there would be more information and more decisions to be made after the surgery. Still, one might consider doing something other than going off to spend the morning in an isolated, windowless office in a funeral home two days before cancer surgery. Surgery. Such a sterile word for what was going to happen to me. They were going to cut off a body part.

Having just come off Breast Cancer Awareness Month, I was sick to death of all things pink. And boobs and boobies and knockers and tits. *"Save the ta-tas!"* It was all a bit too much for me just then. I wanted it all to go away.

After work, I headed to the hospital for my pre-op tests. A lung X-ray, blood work, and an EKG all went well in the hands of the very capable nurses and technicians. We were told to arrive by 10:00 a.m. on Wednesday for my 12:05 p.m. surgery, a seemingly arbitrary time at which the scalpel would do its work.

On Tuesday morning, I awoke with the strangest feeling. The last full day with my right breast. I went to work, then spent the afternoon catching up on some writing. It was a day like many other days, but I couldn't pass by a mirror without staring at my chest. I did the same thing when I was 12 and those same breasts were beginning to sprout at last.

Then, it was all about anticipation. How big would they be? What will I look like?

Now all I wanted was to soak it in, to capture the feeling of having a normal chest and hold on to it forever. I had many of the same questions, but with an entirely different mindset. What would I look like tomorrow? Next week? Next year? More importantly, would I would be lucky enough to still be here at all?

At 12, I could put something under my shirt to see how I would look with breasts. At 51, there was nothing I could do to see how I would look minus one.

Liz was so distracted that she decided to take Wednesday afternoon off from school and work. She wanted to wait for Jim to call and tell her that surgery was over. She was worried about him, too, picturing him pacing around in the waiting room all alone. I shared that concern.

David and Tommy both called to chat and I felt, not for the first time, that I'm the most fortunate mother in the world for having such loving children.

So, what do you do on the eve of a mastectomy? Conduct a photo shoot, of course. We wanted to take advantage of this final opportunity to capture the image of me the way I was. It's a shame that I was still bruised from the biopsy, but that's part of the authenticity of the moment.

I suppose the pre-mastectomy photo shoot is a fairly common event. When I look at those photos now, I am not saddened by the loss. On the contrary, it makes me smile. I'd have to say that breasts look better in pairs, but old Pristine is holding her own.

It's not only my chest that has changed since those photos were taken; it's all of me. My hair, my eyebrows and lashes, the fine lines around my eyes. I look so different. Yet, if you look directly into my eyes, I'm not so very different. That night, I stared confidently and directly into the lens, as if to communicate with Future Ann and let her know I was strong enough. Future Ann can look right back now. If she could, she'd tell Past Ann that life is pretty darned good.

Before retiring to bed, I wrote a brief, but heartfelt love note to Jim and placed inside his dresser drawer, just in case...

We slept peacefully throughout the night. We woke up early on Wednesday morning and lounged under the covers, holding each other for a long time. I felt relaxed and thankful in our cozy state. That is the stuff of life and I soaked it in for as long as I could.

When we could stall no longer, I got up and showered, offering a silent farewell to Pristine's twin.

Then the time for sentiment was over and I resolved to get on to the business of saving my life. Time to close up that filing cabinet again.

We set off for the hospital at about 9:30 a.m. We didn't even have time to pull out our Kindles before we were ushered inside. I was hustled into a hospital gown and introduced all around. It hasn't always been my experience with health care, but at this hospital, on this day, every nurse, every technician, and every staff member we crossed paths with was professional and caring. They didn't treat me as a case; they treated me as a person who was about to undergo a profound life change.

We had an interesting nurse who told us about her own mastectomy 14 years earlier. She was quite a talker, filling every void with tales of her hardscrabble life. Everyone has a story to tell and there are times when we need to hear them as much as they need to be told.

At 10:00 a.m., someone showed up with a wheelchair of monumental proportions. Seriously? You couldn't find one that wouldn't make me look so pitiful? You could have fit two of me in that thing. The footrests were ridiculously far apart, forcing me into a very unladylike position. How terribly undignified! I repositioned myself to one side of my new vehicle and put both feet on a single footrest. With a blanket covering my legs, I was a bit less conspicuous and ready for the ride over to the nuclear medicine department.

The hospital was bustling with activity. Doctors and nurses passing each other in the hallways, people in wheelchairs being pushed to and from procedures, medical chatter filling the air. The bright lights and unfamiliar sounds, combined with the movement of the wheelchair, sent me into sensory overload. It was just shy of an out-of-body experience.

Once at my destination, I was to receive some type of dye that would help the surgeon do her thing with my sentinel lymph nodes. In breast cancer, the sentinel lymph nodes are the first to which cancer is likely to spread from the primary tumor. This information is needed to stage the cancer and to help plan treatment.

The dye would not be given intravenously – it would be injected directly into my still sore right breast. The fun never ends.

I was positioned flat on the table as a doctor used a needle to pierce my skin and inject the dye into four separate locations around my areola. An additional eight injections were scattered throughout my breast. It was not a good feeling, but the doctor went out of his way to be nice and performed his task with speed and precision. He even apologized as he realized he would be injecting right into the bruise left by the biopsy. It was one of those, "I can't believe this is actually happening to me" moments.

Lucky Pristine. She can just sit over there and relax. That poor right breast is probably thrilled to go, just to end the torture, I thought. I felt terrible that the sting of the needles would be the last thing it would ever feel. I was assigning emotion to my breast, even as I realized how ridiculous it was.

Then it was back into the oversized wheelchair for another spin down the hallways.

After another waiting period, Dr. M arrived and greeted us with her customary hugs. She took extreme caution to mark the correct side of my chest, her attention to detail and bedside manner of tremendous comfort.

Jim and I got to spend a few more minutes together before it was time for me to head for the operating room. He wanted to move mountains to save me from this, but all he could do at that moment was love me. That's all I needed, anyway.

As I exited the room in my rolling bed, my heart went out to him. I would have the luxury of sleeping through the rest of this ordeal. He had the unenviable task of waiting for word that I was well...or that they'd discovered worse news. His was the more difficult road for the time being.

No matter how close you are as a couple, there are some things you are destined to face on your own. Of the two of us, only Jim would be left standing as his wife was wheeled away, when the only thing he wanted to do – to rescue her – was the one thing he could not do.

In spite of all the people in the room, and of all the people who loved me, I was on my own then. I alone would enter the operating room to put my life in the hands of others and I alone would leave the operating room with one less body part, knowing that was only the beginning of a very uncertain journey.

I had surgeries before, unfortunately, but this would be the first time I expected to wake up with so many questions yet to be answered. For everyone's sake, I hoped the surgery would be over quickly.

We'd already survived a lot, and we managed to keep "living, laughing, and loving despite MS." Would we manage to do the same despite cancer?

The surgery team did a thorough job of going over the pre-surgery checklist, even soliciting my confirmation on the purpose of the surgery and which breast was targeted. What must it feel like to be on the medical team, to have someone's life in your hands, I wondered. What thoughts run through your mind before performing a life-changing surgery like removal of a breast?

The lights were blinding, causing me to squint. I was

shivering despite the two warm blankets they placed over my body. Then somebody mentioned they were about to inject something into my IV that would put me to sleep and the next thing I remember, they were telling me to wake up.

Part seven of the HBO miniseries, "John Adams," depicted Adams' daughter having a mastectomy without benefit of anesthesia. The reenactment was excruciating to watch. How must it have felt, in those days, to have breast cancer? What was it like to be awake during a mastectomy? It was difficult to watch. The scene ended, but I couldn't shake the image or the feelings it provoked within me, yet I had no idea I would ever have breast cancer.

It's a wonderful thing, that miracle called anesthesia. The next few hours in the recovery room are forever lost in the post-surgical haze. I recall realizing that the surgery was over and my breast was gone, that I was happy to be alive, and I'd see Jim soon. I was in little pain and my spirits were good, but my world was pleasantly foggy. I knew I was off, but I was okay with that. I wasn't all that anxious to come back to reality.

How much time passed, I do not know, when I felt myself being wheeled away. The blurry forms who rolled me along could have been anybody and they could have been rolling me anywhere. I could be in a horror movie, and they're taking me to a torture chamber, or maybe I'll wake up in the morgue. No, I'm not dreaming. I'm still in the hospital. I am awake.

As the bed made its way through the halls, I stared at the lights, the ceiling tiles, and the walls as if they were the most interesting things I'd ever seen. I didn't know where to look or how to feel. Should I smile?

Somebody mentioned they were bringing me to my room in the hospital's oncology wing. The oncology wing. Such a serious-sounding wing. It's a place where lives are saved, but sad things happen there, too.

As the foot of my bed reached the doorway, one of the nurses said, "Do you remember this guy?"

The world is a very fuzzy place when I'm not wearing my contact lenses or eyeglasses, but I recognized Jim by the color of his shirt and pants and by his familiar movements. My rock, at last. The fog thinned and I smiled in his direction. I immediately felt him relax. We were together again, I was alive, and part one of treatment was over. Shouldn't we fist bump or something?

When the bed was all the way in the room, Jim inched closer, saying, "I brought this specialist in to see you."

Oh, no. Why do I need a specialist, I wondered. A very tall, thin man stepped out from behind Jim. In the blur that is my nearsighted world, the man looked a lot like my son, David, but even through the haze I knew that could not be so.

The man said hello and darned if he didn't sound like David, too. I must be on some mighty powerful drugs, I thought. He drew nearer, not walking, but floating as one does in a dream, and then I felt his presence. It *was* David! How was that possible? He couldn't be here!

"David?" He leaned in for a gentle hug. "David!"

Jim explained that after I was wheeled off to surgery, he headed toward the waiting room, expecting to spend the next few hours in solitude. As he reached for the door handle, a young man reached for it, too, offering to open it for him. Looking up, it took a moment to register exactly who that young man was. When someone is out of time and place, it takes a minute or two for your brain to put the pieces together. David timed it all so perfectly!

It was my sister's 50th birthday party. She thought she was going out to dinner with a few people, but a dozen or so greeted her with shouts of "surprise!" Then I entered the room, while Jim remained hidden around the corner. I walked up to her and said, "Hello. I'll be your waitress tonight. What can I get you to drink?" At first, she didn't look up as she gave me her drink order.

"I'm sorry. I didn't get that," I said.

She looked up at me and repeated her order. Then she paused as she scanned my familiar face. For a moment, she looked confused, as if she didn't believe her own eyes. Then she knew. "Ann? Ann! What are you doing here?" She didn't expect to see me 500 miles from home.

Jim entered the room and we let everyone in on the second surprise. My brother pulled off a good one. It was hugs all around.

I was elated to learn that Jim didn't have to sit and wait for news all by himself after all. What a relief that must have been! David took time away from work to fly in to be with us on this important and emotional day. It wasn't the first time he pulled off a surprise visit, and, knowing him, it probably wouldn't be the last. It was definitely the most appreciated.

They both stayed with me for a few hours. I remember that we had a lovely time, although details elude me still. David politely excused himself each time the nurses came in to check on my surgical site or take my vitals. Jim always remained, watching with a careful eye.

The postoperative blur continued, but I gathered that the operation was a success. Dr. M believed she removed all the cancer cells and saw no evidence that it had invaded the chest wall. Hallelujah!

As dinnertime rolled around, my two guardians worked it out so that David would stay by my side and Jim would go home, grab a bite to eat, and regroup. It was a break he hadn't expected, though I'm sure it was a welcome one. Jim came back later to say goodnight and they departed together, leaving me to rest.

The rush I get when my kids visit always helped me deal with MS, and David's surprise helped me deal with recovery from this surgery as well. It was just the lift I needed.

Oh, those hospital nights. When you need nothing more than rest, you just can't get it. I was awakened every two hours for maintenance to the drip hanging out of my right side. Then there were the usual blood pressure and temperature checks and antibiotics that needed to be pushed through the IV. Had it not been for the fact that I had a mid-level migraine, the night would have been a lot easier. I couldn't wait to get out of there so I could sleep for real.

About 27 hours after walking into the hospital, I walked out, flanked by my husband and son, wearing my new gray fleece pants and red zip up hoodie.

Clipped to the inside of my tee shirt was the drainage tube, held in place against my skin by a few stitches. The long tube ended in a drainage bulb to capture blood and other fluids. The tube would stay in place for a minimum of one week, during which we were to strip and clean it several times a day, measuring and recording the amount of liquid captured.

On the ride home, the seatbelt's shoulder harness crossed right over my surgical site, so I had to hold it away from my body. I hoped that discomfort wouldn't last long.

I hadn't received, or simply didn't remember receiving information about purchasing a special camisole that had a pocket for the drainage bulb and would make things a bit more comfortable. In the end, it didn't seem to matter much, as the tube would be out in fairly short order, anyway. It was nothing a tee shirt/hoodie combo couldn't handle.

Still to come would be the removal of the bandages on my chest, an event I wasn't looking forward to. More importantly, in a few days, we would have the pathology report on the lymph nodes and the cancer would be staged. That would be very useful to the oncologist who was to formulate the next phase of treatment. Many questions remained, but we were relieved to have this first part of treatment behind us.

I spent much of the next day sitting around and chatting with David. Jim stayed close by, but was able to get a little work done, too.

David had to head home early Friday morning. Our visit was all too brief, but it helped Jim and me to feel less isolated during those strange days. I know the trip probably caused him great inconvenience, but he's an incredible son who did me a world of good. What wonderful talks we had and how special he made me feel!

There was a catch in my throat and a tear in my eye as I watched him drive away. With his departure went our pleasant distraction from what was still to come. We were, once again, on our own.

It's one thing to explain the physical process of mastectomy and recovery. It's quite another to find the words to express the emotional process. We each deal with things according to our own life experiences, our own hopes and fears. I know what it's like to lose a breast, but I would not presume to know how other women deal with that loss.

Indeed, my own processing of this event was a product of my age (51) and place in life (happily married, childbearing years behind me, MS). The cosmetics of it all, while not unimportant to my self-image, didn't cause turmoil or depression. I was confident in the decision to have the mastectomy, as well as the decision not to seek reconstructive surgery in the near future.

The full support of my husband certainly made my ordeal easier to bear than it might have been otherwise. Still, the emotional processing of losing a breast does not end after the surgery.

The next step would be the unveiling of my new figure. I was surprised, and somewhat horrified, to learn that we were expected to remove the bandages from my chest at home. These are the things you don't think about until they happen to you, or to someone close to you. I simply hadn't given it any thought.

It was suggested that I take a shower first to allow the

water to loosen the bandages. In the shower was as good a place as any. I wanted to be alone, anyway.

Being the pragmatic sort, I set aside two hours of crying time and not a moment more. Crying can be a useful tool to release emotions. I have no problem with appropriate crying, but the trick is not to allow it to continue beyond its usefulness.

Although we'd done some online sleuthing and saw photos of mastectomy patients, I wasn't at all certain what I would look like just 48 hours after surgery.

Before stepping into the shower, I washed my face and put my contact lenses in so I could see clearly. Showering after a mastectomy requires some thought, due to the drain hanging out of your side. As suggested by the doctor, Jim made a necklace of sorts out of string so we could hang the drain from it while I showered. It was an awkward experience and it made me feel somewhat vulnerable.

I washed first, allowing water to saturate the bandages. Finally, I began gingerly pulling away at the edges, expecting it to hurt. It didn't; in reality, I had no feeling at all in the area. A large swath of my chest was numb.

No photo could have prepared me for the shock of looking down and seeing nothing where a breast used to be. My beautiful little breast was replaced with a long line of stitches, beginning in the center of my chest and reaching to a rather concave area under my arm. It appeared to be a good outcome, considering the potential for problems. The doctor was able to use dissolvable stitches and it actually looked better than one might expect. It was more about what was missing that caused me to gasp. Despite some swelling, the right side of my chest was frighteningly flat and thin. It would take some time for my brain to adjust to this new image.

I couldn't yet remove the second bandage that was placed over the drain, as tears began to cloud my vision. I heard a faint, almost foreign whimpering sound coming from somewhere inside me. The file cabinet was spilling its contents.

Jim was respecting the space I'd asked for, but listened for my reaction and any hint that he was needed. He entered the bathroom, asking if I needed help. Should I cover myself? Should I hide? I cringed as he pulled aside the white shower curtain. My husband was about to see my new physical state for the first time. I never felt so exposed and naked, a stranger in my own body.

I turned to face him and he didn't miss a beat or avert his eyes. He looked directly at my chest and underarm, then into my eyes, without the slightest hint of revulsion or disgust. A slight wave of nausea came over me and I had to make use of the shower chair we bought back when my MS was raging. Jim helped me remove the bandage around the drain site.

After a few minutes, the whimpering was over and he assisted me out of the shower. There. It was done. We both saw my body. There would be no reason to hide on that day or ever.

The post-op instructions recommended air-drying, so I took that to heart. I wrapped a large bath towel around my waist and propped myself up on the end of the bed, directly in front of the dresser mirror. I was not going to shy away from my own appearance. I would own it. I stared at myself, knowing this was probably the worst it would ever look. The swelling would go down, the stitches would be removed, and the drainage tube was a temporary annoyance. Even the scarring would fade a little over time. Pristine was looking absolutely regal, secure in her appearance, even without her twin. A breast for a life. Not a bad trade at all. Total crying time? About 10 minutes.

Even though a nurse had schooled Jim in the process of stripping and emptying the drain and bulb, I decided to do it myself. I had no trouble reaching around and getting the job done, so it seemed rather silly to have Jim do it. Believe me, although he was prepared to do what was necessary, he was relieved that he didn't have to. His caregiver role turned out to be less than anticipated. I didn't need or want his help with tube maintenance, but he willingly took on most of my physical household chores for a few weeks.

I had a prescription for a strong pain reliever in hand when I was discharged from the hospital, but after taking one that day, I felt no need to take more. Perhaps that was because of all the medical problems I'd previously experienced with MS, along with a long history of migraines. I tend to rate all pain on the migraine scale, and this pain was not in that league. My chest ached but it was tolerable and I wanted to keep my head clear.

I spent a large part of Friday afternoon on the phone with family. It wasn't until after dinner that I began to feel fatigued. So much happened in such a short period that fatigue was not surprising. I was trying to alternate between moving around appropriately for mild exercise and resting...and spending quality time with Jim.

My sense of self would not change unless I permitted it to. I knew I would still feel feminine and – dare I say it – sexy. That's right. I still felt sexy. I was still me!

The pathology report wasn't due for a few days, but Dr. M called while it was "hot off the press," bless her heart. She had good news to share and didn't want to wait. Confirming what she observed during surgery, the report showed that my lymph nodes were absolutely clear, as was my chest wall. She staged me at IIA, which was better than she had anticipated, and sweet music to our ears.

That IIA staging was because the tumor was larger than two centimeters across, but had not spread to the lymph nodes or to distant sites, as far as anyone could tell. In an odd twist, I learned that I actually had five sentinel lymph nodes while most people have one or two. I've always got to be different. All five were removed.

When you have lymph nodes removed from under your arm, you must be forever on the alert for lymphedema, a blockage of the lymph vessels that drain fluid from the tissues. This can cause chronic swelling of the arm. For that reason, you must avoid stressing that arm, and that includes using blood pressure cuffs, injections, and IVs. Good thing my other arm wasn't affected.

Later, when we received a copy of the pathology report, it was another visual confirmation of just how serious this cancer was.

The most frightening finding for me was that it was "lymphovascular invasion positive," meaning the cancer had acquired the genetic mutation it needed to create its own blood vessels. This meant that the tumor might have already begun to spread cancer cells to other parts of my body, signaling the need for aggressive treatment. It sounded monstrous, indeed, like in those alien movies when some creature from beyond inhabits a human body.

We also learned that the tumor measured just short of three centimeters and, rather than calling it "moderately-differentiated," it was now listed as "poorly-differentiated" and with a "high mitotic rate." That's the rate at which cells divide. The higher the rate, the more aggressive the cancer. Mine was a grade three tumor. On a scale of one to three, that's the least desirable grade.

The days that followed brought extreme fatigue. While I experienced surprisingly little pain, there was a great deal of discomfort and many weird sensations emanating from my chest and arm.

When I moved a certain way, it sent a tugging or prickly feeling to my upper arm and my nonexistent breast and nipple. Sometimes it felt like an electrical charge. The feeling was very powerful and if I didn't look down, I felt as if my right breast was still there. Even so, my surface skin was, for the most part, without feeling. I'd heard about missing limbs causing phantom feelings, but for whatever reason, it didn't occur to me that it would be true of a breast. To this day, as far as my brain is concerned, that breast is present and accounted for.

My thoughts turned once again to surgery, as I worked

through my feelings about breast reconstruction. Since Dr. M had strongly advised holding off on thoughts of reconstruction for a while, not getting that process started during the mastectomy surgery meant that it would be a bit more involved should I ever change my mind. After some research on reconstruction, the risks and expense began to sound more and more unappealing. I couldn't help but picture a bag of some foreign material placed underneath my stretched skin. I have no doubt that I'd look at the whole thing differently if I were younger or in different circumstances, but a good prosthetic would probably be enough for me.

This is a choice each woman must make on her own. There is no one-size-fits-all answer to something as personal as mastectomy and breast reconstruction. There is no right or wrong choice, only our individual choice.

As for Jim, the answer was clear. "If you do consider reconstruction, just know that you will be doing it for yourself, not for me, because I think you look beautiful just the way you are."

Wow.

CHAPTER 6

Transitions

Sunday, November 14 marked one month since that moment I discovered a lump in my breast. Already the landscape of my body was forever altered.

Was it possible that I'd already made my peace with it? I was certainly not in a state of denial, but I was strangely at ease with the changes and conscious of the fact that there would be many more. After my morning shower, I took a long, hard look at chest. Even if you're not large-breasted, losing one breast changes the landscape around a much larger area than you would think.

As Jim entered the room, I felt no anxiety about my nakedness. I was comfortable with a fluffy white towel wrapped around my waist, the drain, its bulb, and the adhesive strips still in place. They were but temporary inconveniences that would be gone and forgotten before I knew it.

I read that many women have difficulty showing their husbands their chest after mastectomy, some saying they were never able to do so. I can't imagine living like that. There was a new physical me, and we had no intention of running from that.

Recovery from the surgery was going well for the most part, with fatigue being the most difficult symptom.

A few days after surgery, a coughing fit that came out of nowhere woke me up at 1:30 a.m. The coughing caused pain at the surgical site. I couldn't get it under control, so Jim got up and made some soothing caffeine-free green tea for me.

After awhile, the cough was better, but I couldn't get back to sleep. I ended up on the sofa about 3:00 a.m., hoping to be lulled to sleep by mindless television.

Smokey couldn't seem to get enough of me, so I had to use a pillow as body armor. Why are cats so in need of affection when you don't want them around and so aloof when you do? I sure didn't want her touching my chest, and it would have been extremely unpleasant indeed if she had been able to get to the tubing coming out of my side.

I never did fall back into restful slumber, instead fading into and out of sleep. I was plagued by visions or dreams; I was never sure which, as the line between wakefulness and sleep can be ever so blurry when you're exhausted. Everywhere I looked, people with saws were walking toward me, steadily and purposefully aiming for my chest.

My tormentors were not doctors. They wore work pants and big work boots, but they had no faces. Chain saws, table saws, hand saws, hack saws. I could hear the unsettling whirring of engines, the horrible clanging of blades, and imagined those sharp blades making impact with my chest. I could feel them hitting my skin again and again.

I was able to squelch my troubled thoughts during the day, but the darkness of night offered no such control. Those nightmarish visions, even in the light of this day, I cannot erase from my mind.

Although I wouldn't be working at the funeral home until Dr. M gave her approval, I was back on track with my writing clients. It's amazing the difference a few days can make.

As Jim and I admired a delivery of the get-well flowers that arrived, tears sprung to my eyes so quickly that even I was stunned. I didn't feel the emotion coming on.

I wasn't sure if I was touched by the gesture or sad. Jim sweetly comforted me and my little emotional display dissipated as quickly as it appeared. Moments later, wrapped in his sweet embrace, I felt as beautiful as a fairytale princess.

My emotions came in waves, forcefully rushing toward the surface and gently falling away again.

What Jim and I shared, both emotionally and physically, remained intact. He showed no hint of sorrow at my missing breast. I understood that in time, those feelings could change, but there was no need to dwell on that. Pristine was beautiful, and a prosthesis would balance her off nicely after the healing process was complete. I was alive, gloriously alive, and that was enough for the moment.

Cancer. Perhaps not the certain death sentence it once was, but it's still a tough topic. Some people don't want to talk about it, some don't know how, and some live in fear of it. So, what should you say to someone who has breast cancer? Well, I'll start with what you shouldn't say.

Don't immediately launch into a tale about the horrible side effects of treatment, question her choices, or list names of people who died of cancer. Nor should you downplay the serious nature of the beast. A few simple words of support or a hug will do. Really. It's probably better to ask questions about how someone is feeling than to offer advice based on what you've read or heard or assume she may be feeling. Follow her lead.

Now I don't possess a golden tongue and am guilty of my fair share of gaffes, so I cut a lot of slack for people who do the same. However, I do have a few suggestions.

Let me begin with this: Please don't tell a person with breast cancer, *"Just be grateful you don't have (insert any other form of) cancer."*

I can't even count the number of times I've been told this and I resented it each time. Of course I was grateful. I don't go around telling people with the flu to be grateful they aren't having a heart attack. Of *course* it could have been worse – for any one of us on any day – and that means you, too. Why would anyone assume I'm not grateful? I was also grateful that I wasn't being stabbed in the eye with a hot poker or having my ass lit on fire, but I still had cancer. It's still life altering and life threatening. People die from it. It's what I was dealing with at the time, regardless of how many other horrible things could have happened.

It's the same kind of logic I heard when I was diagnosed with MS. *"Oh, you're so lucky it's not ALS (or muscular dystrophy or some other disease)."* While it may be helpful to point this out to an overly dramatic, die-hard "woe is me" type, it is not helpful to the average person with a level head. Think carefully before comparing diseases. Better yet, just don't compare diseases.

The breast cancer awareness campaign has to be one of the most successful campaigns ever. Unfortunately, pink fatigue has led people to believe breast cancer so common or so curable that it's not such a big deal anymore. After all, look at all those smiling women wearing pink and running marathons!

Maybe you know someone who had "precancerous" cells or a lumpectomy for stage I or even stage 0 breast cancer. Perhaps treatment for a slow-growing variety was minimal and recovery fairly short. But all breast cancers are not alike. This is an important detail that may have escaped your notice, as it had mine before it hit home.

In recent decades, treatment for breast cancer has greatly improved survival rates, but despite all things pretty in pink, breast cancer can – and does – kill. Naturally, survival rates depend on a great many factors, including age, overall health, stage at diagnosis, treatment choices, etc.

In addition to the obvious health problem, the financial considerations, especially if you are uninsured or under-insured, create tremendous stress. Employment and family strains add to the mix. Breast cancer, no matter what stage or type, is not all ribbons and bows.

Back in the Things Could Always Be Worse Department, someone told me, *"At least it's not an arm or a leg or something you really have to use."* Exactly how is one supposed to respond to that? I know it was an attempt to make me feel better, but I'm still quite attached to all my body parts, including my breasts, thank you. The fact that other body parts weren't being cut off was definitely a plus, but not really relevant to the situation at hand. Unless, of course, I had the option to choose one part over another...

Okay, good news for all the small-breasted women of the world. Fear not. After all, *"You're small! It could have been worse!"* I kid you not. Someone actually said that to me. I was speechless.

I know I'll get some disagreement on this, but one of the most vexing of all comments is something along the lines of, *"It's all mental. If you decide to beat it, you will."*

During the course of 10 months of treatment and beyond, I got that one a lot, both from people I knew and from complete strangers, many prompted only by the sight of my bald head.

I get what they were trying to say, I really do. I believe wholeheartedly in a mind/body connection. I believe our frame of mind can change a great deal about how we feel on a daily basis, and helps us to triumph over obstacles great and small. It can make all the difference in how we fight disease and in how we enjoy life.

The ability to hold on to positive feelings – to put fear aside and to truly live in the moment – is what sustains me and many others who have serious health problems. The mental component is a vital key to living each day to the fullest and not becoming all about a disease.

What I don't like about the whole positive attitude mantra is the insinuation that in order to have a positive attitude you must suppress all feelings of frustration, anger, or fear. Those emotions don't make you a negative person. They make you human. You have to be honest with yourself and with others if you want to work through those feelings and move on. You can explore the full range of human emotion and still be a positive person.

Anyone who insists that you wear a happy face every moment of the day isn't doing you any favors. As far as I can see, that's more helpful to them than to you. Less for them to deal with.

I embraced the idea of positive attitude many years ago. For me, it's a lifestyle choice. However, I do not believe that mental attitude is enough. You have to channel those positive thoughts into action by making healthy lifestyle decisions and seeking appropriate medical care. There are other forces at work, too, and whether we care to admit it or not, some things are totally beyond our control.

I cannot accept that people who succumb to cancer or other sometimes treatable diseases did so because they had the wrong attitude or didn't try hard enough, and it's a horrible burden to place on them and on their surviving loved ones. If frame of mind is all it takes, none of us needs to die – ever.

Don't deny the negative but focus on the positive. Acknowledge the worst-case scenario, but aim for the best. That's our philosophy, anyway.

I take comments like these with a grain of salt, understanding that sometimes words just tumble out before the speaker can fully appreciate their impact. We've all done it at one time or another. My own foot is well acquainted with the inside of my mouth.

Fortunately, I've also been the recipient of an outrageous number of kindnesses and comforting words. Trust me on this point – the most effective and appreciated gestures are the simple ones.

One week following surgery, it was time for my post-op visit with my surgeon. Dr. M was very pleased with my quick recovery. She also removed a buildup of fluid from my chest. It was very strange to watch her insert a needle into what should be a very tender area and feel absolutely nothing. She also removed the last of the adhesive strips. The fluids collected from the drain had declined enough to warrant removal of the tube. She removed the stitches and, with a deep breath and a pull, the tube was out. Thankfully, it only took a few seconds. What a relief to be freed from my personal ball and chain! She told me to begin massaging the skin on my chest to keep it from "sticking." It hurt a little, but I knew it was just another temporary discomfort.

I quizzed her about breast cancer risk for Liz. She told me that my daughter is definitely at increased risk of breast cancer because I had it. I knew that, but I didn't enjoy hearing it. She told me that Liz should be self-aware, perform self-exams, and perhaps begin mammograms at age 35. She pointed out that those recommendations were subject to change because technology will probably be in a whole different place in another decade.

As well as I was doing, she advised me to continue to stay home from work until the Monday after Thanksgiving. She also cautioned that I might begin to feel increased pain over the next few weeks due to fluid retention and swelling. I was scheduled to follow up again in two weeks.

After leaving her office, we stopped by the local medical supply store. While I would not be able to be measured for a prosthesis for at least three months during the healing process, I did have the go-ahead to wear a "foamie," a lightweight piece of foam that can be pinned behind the cup of a bra. At least I could balance out my chest and get beyond the oversized hoodies I'd been wearing.

Things were looking up.

CHAPTER 7

Bringing in the Big Guns

With round one behind us and recovery well underway, it was time to meet with my oncologist, Dr. G. I heard his name before, but couldn't immediately put my finger on where or why.

Jim and I had plenty of time to anticipate the appointment, but we were still a bit on edge. This doctor would be a vital part of my treatment for a long time to come. If he was anything like "a" doctor, I was going to have to find someone else.

The appointment desk set aside a full hour for this introductory visit and we would have plenty of ground to cover. It was time to find out what round two had in store for us, time to formulate the long-term plan to beat cancer.

When we walked into the outer office, we were stunned by the size and scope of the operation and the number of people in the waiting room. The very efficient receptionist was able to field phone calls, pass out clipboards of paperwork, and keep everyone and everything organized, and she did it all with a smile. That woman deserves a medal.

Once we made it back to the doctor's office, it didn't take us long to realize that good luck had found us yet again. Dr. G possessed a great deal of empathy, patience, and a willingness to answer questions in depth. Like Dr. M, he didn't hold back on hard realities, but was reassuring nonetheless.

He began with a thorough explanation of triple-negative breast cancer and some unknowns about treatment. He told us there was a good chance that all the cancer was removed during surgery and that I'd already beaten it. How about that? It was one of those good news/bad news things because it was impossible to know how many microscopic cancer cells may have been left behind. If any did remain, they could be in my breast tissue or already working their way to distant parts of my body where they could lie dormant for years or begin their quest for dominance right away.

Triple-negative breast cancer responds well to chemotherapy, so it was very likely that I would finish chemo cancer-free, he told us.

Taking into account my medical history and the pathology of the tumor, his plan called for 16 rounds of chemotherapy. The first four rounds would be given at three-week intervals and would consist of two chemo drugs – Adriamycin and Cytoxan. Chemotherapy doesn't always cause hair loss, but that cocktail came with a 100 percent chance of baldness. Oh, well.

That would be followed by 12 rounds of Taxotere, given once a week. This would, indeed, be a very long haul. Was I happy to be pouring harsh drugs into my body week after week? Most certainly not. But with everything we'd learned about triple-negative breast cancer, we felt strongly that it had to be done.

After discussing the basics of chemotherapy, Dr. G offered the possibility of a clinical trial. It would involve a lengthier treatment time, we'd have less information about the actual medications I would receive, and I'd need extra tests to follow my progress.

Then there would be additional concerns about which treatments my health insurance would pay for and which it would not, but the doctor's office would help us navigate those waters. The threat of an MS relapse could only complicate matters. We discussed the pros and cons at length and declined.

Clinical trials are enormously helpful to researchers, but

we didn't feel prepared to risk my treatment so early on. Just as important, we didn't want the added burden of worrying about what my health insurance may or may not cover. We needed a clearer roadmap than that.

Dr. G actually seemed pleased with our choice, saying it probably wasn't right for me, anyway, but that he wanted us to come to that decision ourselves. He would hold off making a recommendation about radiation therapy until we neared the end of chemotherapy.

As he spoke, it dawned on me why his name was familiar. I'd seen his signature on death certificates at the funeral home. Oncologists sign their fair share of those. Would his name someday appear on my death certificate? I shuddered at the thought and shook it off.

My first treatment was scheduled for the morning of December 1. Tommy would be arriving for a visit the evening before, so I set the appointment for early in the morning. I didn't want to tie up a full day, nor did I want him to have to sit through my inaugural chemotherapy with me. Besides, Jim said he wanted to be there. Actually, he planned on being there for every single one of them.

My second session was already on the schedule for December 23, when Liz would be visiting. It promised to be an eventful month.

Thanksgiving is a time for large family gatherings and giving thanks for all our good fortune. We would not have the family gathering, but we had much thankfulness in our hearts.

We prepared our little feast together, expressed our thanks, watched a movie, and played Wii. Just the two of us. A delicious, romantic Thanksgiving it was, too.

By Friday, our thoughts turned, once again, to health. Well before my MS went into this lengthy remission, I'd stopped seeing a neurologist and stopped getting MRIs and other expensive MS-related tests. Life had gotten far too complicated and my condition only seemed to get worse. Certainly, it was a stressful situation. I still saw our general physician and took my disease-modifying MS medication, but I felt better with less medical intrusion in my daily life. I never really knew if the medication was working or not, and perhaps it was time to reconsider my options.

Should I continue taking this powerful medication every day now that my body was about to endure chemotherapy, too? We briefly discussed going back to my former neurologist for his opinion. Maybe he could do an MRI, and then follow me after going off the medication. It didn't take me long to nix that idea.

I didn't want to face life that way – bouncing among a surgeon, a general physician, an oncologist, and a neurologist – and all the additional tests that would be required. If I let myself become a full-time patient, everything would unravel and it would kill my spirit. Less is often more, I knew.

I'd been injecting myself every day for seven years, but until the seventh year, the relapses continued to worsen. Despite the remission, I wanted to stop putting this substance in my system. Stopping could not kill me, but the long-term effect was a great unknown. It was a chance I was willing to take.

It wasn't a decision I took lightly and I do not offer any opinion as to whether or not people with MS should take disease-modifying drugs, or which ones they should take. MS is an extremely variable disease and each person, along with his or her own doctor, must choose the most promising course. For me, it seemed like a good time to change things up.

I contacted the doctor at Johns Hopkins who diagnosed my MS in 2004. He had no objection to my plan to stop taking the medication while on chemotherapy. He suggested I revisit the issue when cancer treatment was complete. At our next appointment, we had an in-depth discussion with Dr. G, who found no reason to disagree.

When the call came that my "foamy" had arrived, I wasted no time getting over to the medical supply store to pick it up. After a few weeks of oversized tops and a misshapen appearance, it would be nice to be balanced out again. The foam form was lightweight and could be secured to my bra with a safety pin. It still managed to move around a little, but it was definitely a step in the right direction. A little shift here and a little shift there, and off you go. In a few months, I'd be able to order a good prosthesis and move on.

While at the store, I hesitantly picked out a head covering in anticipation of losing my hair. It would work well enough until I could buy some good hats or a wig. I also received a nice "welcome" gift bag full of cancer patient "goodies." I've long since forgotten what, exactly was in that bag, aside from a pink planning calendar and a very useful lightweight pillow that would hold the seatbelt shoulder harness off my chest until I healed. I wish I'd discovered that trick earlier. As for the calendar, it was the key to keeping everything straight over the next year.

Can you believe there's such a thing as "chemo class?" It makes all the sense in the world. Despite the hour-long session we had with Dr. G, his practice also conducts chemo class for all patients as they begin chemotherapy. It's such a lengthy and consuming process that knowing all you can at the outset would take some of the mystery out of it. We'd come a long way from "a" doctor.

It was a mixed group that showed up for the 8:00 a.m. Monday morning session. Some brought partners, some came alone. The mood was fairly serious. I'd already done my research, but the session would solidify what I knew and hone in on the details I had yet to learn.

According to the nurse who took the lead, since the practice implemented this educational class, they cut down considerably on unnecessary trips to the ER and mountains of patient angst. I could believe it.

The nurse assured us that from that moment forward, we should consider ourselves to be on a 24/7 clock with the doctor's office, meaning that day or night, someone would always be available to answer questions and guide us through our concerns. We were given particulars about the practice and staff and encouraged to become partners in our own treatment. As the months passed, I would discover that those were not empty words.

There are many different chemotherapy drugs. The drugs and dosages are tailored to individual needs and specific medical history. The list of potential side effects is seemingly endless. Some people sail through treatment with little trouble while others suffer many side effects and become quite ill. The plan is always subject to change.

I could expect each session to last anywhere from two to six hours. We received information about how to maintain our health while on chemo, including tips on diet, rest, and exercise, along with strong encouragement to remain active and engaged. "Eat!" they kept telling us. No one ever had to force me to eat and I couldn't believe that would ever become a major problem for me. Boy, was I wrong about that.

We learned simple strategies for coping with side effects of chemo, as well as when and how to reach out for help.

The nurse suggested we visit our local chapter of the American Cancer Society office to say hello and find out what services they provide. Jim and I never actually got around to doing that, as we managed well enough on our own. It was nice to know we had a backup, though.

All in all, it was a good session. I went off to work that morning with my head fairly exploding with new information. The basic feeling I took away was that I was part of the equation and that my questions or concerns would not be dismissed. It never felt that way with MS. At the risk of offending neurologists, they always made me feel like a bother. MS treatment and cancer treatment, at least in my case, were turning out to be very, very different. My heart will always be with people with MS and other chronic, "invisible" conditions.

After class, I headed to the funeral home, my first day back at work since surgery. The gang seemed surprised by how well I looked.

The next evening, Jim and I headed out to the airport to welcome Tommy. My heart warmed at the very sight of him. How handsome, healthy, and confident he looked! A few hours later, settling in on the sofa with some popcorn and TV, all was right with the world. Good medicine.

The first of December was gloomy, quite appropriate for what we were about to do. It was cold, windy, and rainy. Tommy slept in while Jim and I headed to the doctor's office.

We arrived at 9:00 a.m. and settled in the waiting room, each with our new Kindles loaded with reading material. Then we were called in for a health insurance consultation. Now *that's* some scary stuff, causing us to wonder how on earth anyone can afford cancer. The manager was a little confounded by my particular policy, but then again, so were we. To the best of her knowledge, we'd be okay. Good enough for the moment.

Next, it was off to the lab for blood work, something that would be done prior to each session. Unsatisfactory blood work meant that treatment would be delayed, they explained.

Then it was off to the chemo room. There's no way to adequately explain the feeling of walking into that room full of people trying to beat cancer. Even weirder to realize that you are one of them.

We were assigned to nurse Patty, who bore a striking resemblance to Kathy Bates. Not scary Kathy Bates, mind you, but smiley Kathy Bates.

It couldn't have been be more surrealistic if accompanied by a fog machine and the theme music to *The Twilight Zone*. Had this place always existed a mere two miles from my home? The room seemed to continue for a city block, recliners set up in groups of four, several nurses stations, and visitor chairs sprinkling the area. It appeared that about half the patients had visitors with them. Each little section had a TV blaring away. There's always a TV blaring away, isn't there? I like watching TV in my home, but why must we be bombarded with it in so many public places? It definitely got in the way of patient-to-patient conversation.

I didn't yet realize this practice had another chemo room on a floor above this. So many cancer patients. Some receiving treatment, some waiting here, still more in the outer waiting room. Why do we all have cancer?

Do you know that this is going on somewhere near you? That people in your town, on your street, get in their cars in the morning and drive off to this other world where life and death and optimism and resignation coexist? Worse yet, did you know that some people must relocate, or drive for hours to reach such a facility?

What must it take for the nurses to go there, day after day, trying to treat and comfort people of all ages and backgrounds and states of mind?

I can tell you this. After a few sessions, even a place like that can cease to feel strange. The sights and smells and sounds become part of your world. Not that you enjoy them, but you accept them as part of the deal when you agree to do this thing. You hope, with every fiber of your being, that it is but a temporary ritual, and that it is going to prevent you from dying just yet. You know that among the many people sharing this space with you, some are undoubtedly courting death.

The nurse, knowing it was our first session, pointed out the bathrooms and a refreshment area where we could help ourselves to tea, coffee, and juice. We patients were privileged to have cozy recliners and were offered pillows and warm blankets, while our visitors sat in the stiff, upright chairs beside us or lining the wall like soldiers on watch.

As they went through the process of explaining the drugs and potential side effects again, I went into information overload until it all became a mere jumble of words and warnings with no meaning. That's why it's a good idea to have someone with you when you're in a situation like that. What in the world would I have done without my Jim?

Nurse Patty didn't make the vein on the first try (ouch), but the second went well. Before beginning the flow of medication, Patty teamed up with another nurse to execute something similar to a pre-flight checklist. She read my name out loud, then the medication and dosages she was about to administer, matching the information to a stack of paperwork and to my wristband, a procedure they performed before each session. Confirmation being complete, I was officially on chemo. I imagined myself as a runner, crouched into position at the starting line at the moment the gun is fired. Take it easy, this is definitely a marathon.

She wheeled a chair over to my recliner and sat facing me, her hand placed gently on top of my own. Patty explained that during the first session, it is important to closely monitor the patient in case of an allergic reaction. I was a watched pot again. Apparently, a severe allergic reaction can be a life-threatening event during which seconds count. Sometimes, the treatment is as frightening as the disease. Guess that's what you call living life on the edge.

With each change of IV bag came another explanation of the drugs and side effects. There was an anti-nausea medication in the mix, something that makes chemo a much more tolerable experience than it was in previous decades.

Because of my right side mastectomy, all blood work and IV drugs would have to be given through my left arm. In the long term, especially when we moved to the once-a-week schedule, that would be tough on my skinny little arm. They told me that if it became difficult enough, they could implant a chemo port in my chest. Well, now, there's something else to look forward to.

The Adriamycin, we were told, is not-so-affectionately known as the "red devil." So called because of its bright red color, which it is good to know beforehand, will turn your urine red for a few hours.

Near as I could tell, most of the patients were middle-aged or older, some had hair, some donned kerchiefs, caps, or wigs. I was grateful not to see any children present. That would have been hard to take. Some folks looked exhausted, but the mood in the room was surprisingly pleasant.

I wondered about the lives of my fellow patients. Did they have someone to help them through this ordeal? Were they all alone?

There wasn't much privacy in the chemo room and one couldn't help but be drawn in by the drama that surrounded the place. Even though it was a mostly upbeat atmosphere, with smiling nurses and patients who refused to give in to negativity, no one ever forgot why we were all there in the first place.

The man one recliner over quickly captured our attention. When he overheard I was having my very first chemo treatment he turned to me and said, "It's your first time? You're going to be sooo sick..." his words trailing off as if he had so much more to say, but no strength with which to say it. If he hadn't looked so sick himself, I would have thought it was a mean thing to say, but given the circumstances, I couldn't hold it against him. He was obviously suffering with pain and appeared quite weak.

Luke told us he was 47 years old and a tree climber/trimmer by trade. It's not that his name was Luke. I don't actually recall his name. When I remember him, he just seems like a Luke. He was super thin, with a bald head and beard, and loaded with tattoos. He had That Look about him, That Look that told you he had a story to tell.

Pretty much everyone in his family dies of cancer, he told us. He had colon cancer that had spread to his brain. He said he recently had a brain tumor removed and was sent home from the hospital the very next day, as if he still couldn't believe it. He'd also had parts of his intestines removed and was enduring unmanageable pain in his abdomen. He said he hadn't slept in many nights. It was a difficult story to hear.

Things soon took a turn for the dramatic. His friend, who had been seated beside him, excused himself, saying he was thirsty and needed something to drink.

I don't know if it was his friend's departure, or that he just reached the breaking point, but Luke became physically agitated. "I'm in so much pain...nobody's listening to me...I'm in pain over here!"

Two nurses rushed to his side in an attempt to comfort him. He wanted them to commit to some abdominal imaging tests that his insurance company denied. Failing in that, he wanted out. He looked around, perhaps realizing that his friend had not yet returned and he was on his own in this particular struggle.

When things seem so overwhelmingly out of control, it's only natural to seek that thing you believe you can control.

His voice grew louder, capturing the attention of everyone in the vicinity. "I'm done with this! I don't want this anymore!"

I was absolutely horrified by this turn of events during my initiation into chemotherapy. What was I getting into?

One of the nurses returned to her station to contact Luke's doctor. That seemed to placate him for a few moments, allowing him to give in and rest while he waited. Still no sign of the friend.

The doctor arrived in a matter of minutes and explained that the test Luke wanted would not give him the information he sought. The best thing would be to complete the treatment, he was told. "Chemotherapy is your best chance. Let us help you."

His plea fell on deaf ears. The man had suffered, had watched others in his family suffer, and did not want to suffer anymore. It wasn't difficult to understand.

Even though I was new to chemo, I weathered enough health problems in my life to understand what Luke meant. Sometimes, it's enough and it needs to stop, no matter what the price. It was not difficult to envision a scenario in which I would feel the same way.

The doctor left and the nurses put in a final plea. "We want to help you get better. If you leave, you're putting your life in danger."

A few more minutes of heated discussion and Luke declared himself finished with chemo and everything that goes along with it. That's it. Outta here. Goodbye. We, along with the other members of the captive audience, had no choice but to watch events unfold.

Where was that "friend" in this moment of crisis?

The nurses could allow the situation to escalate no further once he made a move to pull the IV out himself. Acknowledging out loud they could not keep him against his will, the nurses gently removed his IV and watched helplessly as he walked away alone, his friend still missing in action.

The nurses exchanged looks that spoke of compassion and frustration and the exhausting nature of an oncology nurse's work. Surely, they knew that there are times when walking away is the right thing to do, but was this one of those times? Was he making the right choice, or was it pain, lack of sleep, and lack of support that prompted his actions?

I could picture the movie scene, Luke taking charge and walking away to die on his own terms to the swell of the music and the tears of the audience.

The room was suddenly quiet as we all digested the real life scene. How many of my fellow patients wanted to follow suit, I wondered. I could imagine us getting up, en masse, and following Luke off into the sunset. How would one know when it was time to stop? Would I?

Judging by the looks on my fellow patients' faces, they were pondering many of the same questions.

Luke was gone and the room changed immediately, as if the lights in the theatre went up and it was time for the audience to leave. The bustling nurses, the constant hum of the televisions, the beeping and booping of medical paraphernalia, a few scattered snores and coughs filled the air as the business at hand resumed. The chemotherapy room never rests.

Jim and I sat, soaking in our new reality, perhaps a bit dazed by the morning's events. The medication continued to drip out of the bags, down the clear tubing, and into my bloodstream. I could only hope it would do what it was supposed to do.

There was a palpable sigh of relief and smiles all around when Luke came sauntering back about a half hour later, still alone, but freshly composed and ready to try again. We wondered what made him come back, but didn't want to ask and risk getting him upset again. I never saw him after that day, but I'll never forget the look in his eyes. The brief crossing of our paths made an impression that would last. Wherever you are, Luke, may peace be with you.

It was amazing to be among these people undergoing such powerful treatment, hopeful, and for the most part, smiling. How many were fighting this thing alone?

Even with Jim to support me, the thoughts that ran loose in my mind, the constant changes and assaults on my body, the questioning of self and how I should be handling those things, those were lone struggles.

We were home by 12:30 p.m., seemingly none the worse for wear. After lunch, Tommy and I spent a wonderful afternoon together. Whether he knew it or not, he was performing the miracle of helping me to live in the moment. I felt amazingly well and energetic. I cooked up a full dinner, ate more than usual, and went to bed feeling great.

I went to work the next morning with no ill side effects. Then I had to stop by the doctor's office for an injection of a drug that is supposed to stimulate production of infection-fighting white blood cells. I would need one injection 24 hours after each chemo session.

Some time later, we would be shocked to discover that my insurer was billed $10,000 for each of these little injections.

Their discount brought it down to about $3,000. They paid 100 percent for the first two I received at the end of 2010, but with a new year came a new $5,000 deductible and we were on the hook. It didn't take long before we met that deductible.

Somewhere along the way, we brought up the subject of sticker shock with a doctor. How can anyone pay $10,000 for a single injection? "Nobody actually pays that price," came the answer. Of course not. It's always got to be more complicated than that. What a system.

The following year, I ran into a similar situation when I ordered a mastectomy bra. The bill I received was significantly higher than the quoted price, and because of my deductible, it was an entirely out-of-pocket expense. When I confronted the company, I was told that they charge a higher price so that when the insurance discount is factored in, they'll receive the amount they wanted in the first place. Give me a break. They shouldn't be allowed to quote a discounted price only to raise it. I wanted the price I was quoted – or they could take their stupid, already worn bra right back. It took about six months to conclude the transaction. What a colossal waste of time and energy.

My short span of thinking I might possibly be a chemotherapy superhero ended abruptly. By evening the powerful drugs hit with a vengeance. I was exhausted and felt like crawling right out of my own suddenly unbearably uncomfortable skin.

Another day and my stomach declared its complete revulsion with anything edible. Just like that, as if someone threw the food switch. Food looked, smelled, felt, and tasted like something that should be marked with a skull and crossbones. Whether attempting to eat or not, my mouth tasted like metal. I brushed my teeth again and again but couldn't get rid of the harsh metallic taste. Even toothpaste tasted like metal.

At age 51, I was having my very first fight with food. If I

could have survived without eating at all, I would have taken that option. My relationship with food wouldn't be the same for a very long time to come.

My tortured sleep was peppered with dreams of disgusting food, food slathered on large platters, food shoved in front of my face. I saw slimy food and food I did not recognize. Food on my chin and food spilling onto my lap. Had I landed in food hell? When I woke up, I wanted all food eliminated from the planet. How can people eat, anyway? What a disgusting habit!

Unpleasant thoughts of food followed me throughout my morning at work. I kept no food in my office, but couldn't get my brain to turn off the food train. I was consumed with negative thoughts about food and its many horrific qualities.

As I prepared dinner that night, I had no desire to eat it. What I did manage to swallow threatened to make the return trip. Remembering advice from chemo class, I turned to plain crackers. Even the chicken soup I made to go with them was a complete turn off. Crackers would sustain me for a few days until I could get regain some level of control.

It was about this time that the news broke that Elizabeth Edwards' breast cancer "was no longer treatable." Although I had no particular kinship with her, it was difficult news to digest just as I was heading down this difficult phase of treatment. Even more disturbing was the announcement just one day later that she was dead.

With Tommy in the house, that news hit a little too close to home. Her children were younger than mine, but I was not ready to leave them yet. Mrs. Edwards was very wealthy and had access to the best health insurance and the best health care money could buy, but her breast cancer could not be stopped. It was yet another example of how deadly this foe can be.

The news reports said that she left letters for her children that included advice on everything from marriage and parenthood to career and religion. I wondered if I should be writing letters or making videos.

What would I tell them, anyway? Much in life depends on context. So many things are not at all what they seem to be and very little is truly black and white in our shades of gray existence.

Empathy is important, and so is kindness. You may enjoy a little good luck along the way, but it's your hard work and determination that'll get you where you want to be. Sometimes, you won't even know where you want to be until you're there. Don't ignore your gut instincts, because they're a product of your life experiences. Life is not fair; so don't expect it to be. It's not fair for anybody else, either. Soak in the simple joys of everyday life and never let the child inside you die. Never pass up the opportunity to make someone else smile. Respect your body and treat it well – it's the only one you'll ever have. Be flexible. Love passionately.

There was still so much to say, so much to experience together. I wanted to be grandmother to their children. I wanted them to be able to share their families with me. I wanted them to have the option of leaning on me through their own childrearing years. The thought process was almost unbearable. I vowed not to let cancer get ahead of me, to be vigilant and as aggressive as it was, to go through the fires of hell if I had to, to get on the other side. I was not ready to leave.

I looked over at Tommy, working on his laptop at the kitchen table, and burst into tears. I didn't want to listen to the news anymore that day.

It felt like only days, but before I knew it, the week was over and it was time for Tommy to board his flight for home. He couldn't possibly know how much his presence helped me to cope with that first chemo session and its aftermath. It's always an emotionally challenging occasion, the day one of my children flies off into the sunset, but those emotions were heightened by my uncertain future. As when David departed, this goodbye was not an easy one.

During the next few days, my teeth began to hurt when I touched them with my toothbrush. Sores began to sprout up on my gums, which started to bleed at the slightest touch. I turned to my chemo class notes again and began using the salt/baking soda/warm water mixture recommended for this problem.

My mirror reflection was changing again. I hadn't felt particularly stressed by the loss of one breast, but my mind was beginning to bounce around, cluttering up my thought process and causing me to criticize my own appearance. Fatigue was unpacking its bags and settling in for the long haul, and the term "chemo fog" began to make sense. A good example of that is evidenced by one sentence from my journal on December 7. It read, "I can't seem to find myself."

My writing was regularly published on Care2.com. Its founder, Randy Paynter, published a piece titled "Shine a Light," the first in a series, and the subject was me. In the article, he wrote of my history with MS and my cancer diagnosis, calling on readers to, "Shine one glorious sunbeam of collective love" on me.

"Please take a moment to send Ann some good thoughts via a brief message in the comments area below. Your words will make a difference, and together we'll show that love is the most powerful force of all."

I must say that it took me a bit by surprise. I couldn't possibly be one of those people you read about in that way. I was flattered, touched, bewildered, and embarrassed all at the same time. Within days, almost 1,000 comments and dozens of emails offered words of kindness and comfort.

When Randy implemented his idea to shine that sunbeam of collective love on an individual, he knew that a few simple words, when spoken or written with a full heart, could make all the difference in the world to the recipient. Imagine the effect when multiplied hundreds of times!

I was deeply moved by the power of love flowing in my direction. And I know from experience that it is every bit as glorious to be part of the sunbeam as it is to receive it.

If you ever get the chance to send some kind words to someone you know, or even someone you don't know, I hope you'll take it.

CHAPTER 8

Back to the Business of Living

You haven't lived until you've been wig shopping. We followed the advice given in chemo class and decided not to wait until I was actually bald. I've never looked good in short hair and I didn't want short hair. It all felt so wrong! The people who ran the store believed in making everything as easy as possible for cancer patients, and that meant no wigs made from real hair, which they warned would require too much care.

What a good time it would have been to break new ground and try a wild new hairdo or go blonde just for the fun of it, but I wasn't feeling adventurous. I wanted to look like me; I wanted to feel like me. Change doesn't always come so easily.

With each wig I tried, the more anxious I became. I solicited Jim's opinion, listened carefully to his critiques and those of the salespeople, and only got more discouraged. Nobody or nothing could accomplish what I wanted because it was not possible. When I finally accepted that no hairpiece could replicate my natural hair, I settled on an acceptable wig. They sent me on my way with a warning: don't bend over hot pots on the stove or near the oven, or you'll damage the wig. Great. That's just the kind of thing that would happen to me. I could just imagine my wig melting on my head as I prepared dinner.

"Il fait chaud!" (It's hot!) My grandmother finally gave in to the heat and humidity of mid-July and removed the thick wig from her head, placing it gingerly on the plastic wig

stand on her mirrored dresser. How strange that she can take her hair off! She looks so funny without it!

When I was a kid, it seemed perfectly normal that my grandmother wore a wig. I assumed that all grandmothers did. She wasn't bald, exactly, but had extremely sparse hair. I don't know how old she was when she started wearing the wig, or why her hair was so thin. We kids found it funny that she took her hair off in the evening and even funnier when she removed it in the middle of a sweltering summer day. I had yet to learn exactly how hot it could get in there!

The wig turned out to be more trouble than it was worth. The artificial hair stuck up stubbornly where it hit the back of my neck, and after a month, the sides began to stick out from my scalp. In retrospect, I should have gone all the way and gotten a better wig with natural hair. Actually, I felt much more comfortable wearing hats. If I had it to do over again, I'd go out and buy a dozen cute hats, adorn myself with big, dangly earrings, and call it a day.

When dealing with MS, I found my health insurance policy difficult to navigate and horribly lacking, despite the high premiums. Far too many many things fell into the "we don't cover that" category. Fortunately for us, things worked differently for cancer treatment.

I learned that a doctor's prescription for a "cranial prosthesis" meant that the purchase of a wig would go toward my deductible, or be covered if the deductible had already been met. Cranial prosthesis – what a phrase. It sounds like I needed a head replacement. I also learned that my chemotherapy would be covered at 100 percent. It felt nothing short of a miracle. Sometimes things do work out.

I began keeping a spreadsheet of cancer-related expenses, with columns for the total cost charged by providers, what my insurer actually paid after discounts, and our out-of-pocket expenses. No one could ever quote a price before a procedure, nor could we ever guess at the insurer discounted price or what our portion would be. When you're trying to stay alive, you just close your eyes and hope it all shakes out okay in the end.

Ten days after that first round of chemo, we suddenly realized we were smack in the middle of the Christmas season. I was in good enough spirits, but it was all I could do to work at the funeral home, keep up with my writing, do the cooking, and help with the chores.

I didn't think I had anything left in me, much less the energy required for decorating the house, addressing greeting cards, and all the other busy work that goes along with the holidays. It seemed like an enormous amount of work.

When Liz announced that she was coming to spend Christmas with us, my attitude flipped and my energy level skyrocketed again. I was three for three – a triple play in the kid department that year. I appreciated the way they tag-teamed me, rather than visiting all at once. It was the perfect way for me to spend some quality time with each of them without overstressing myself physically.

Jim and I dragged out our little Christmas tree and elaborate nativity and spent a day decorating. As it turned out, we were both infused with the holiday spirit. It was just what we needed.

So, the sky was falling. Not really. It was just my hair. I used to joke, back in my Before Cancer days, that if my hair ever began to fall out I'd have trouble noticing. Throughout my life, I've lost great amounts of hair every morning, leaving a messy bathroom floor in its wake. No matter how much fell out, I still had a full crop.

Two weeks after the first chemo, I found out what it's really like to lose your hair. My long, dark locks stuck to my fingers and cluttered up the shower drain. All I had to do was to run my fingers through my hair and – whoops! – there goes another handful.

I could afford to lose quite a bit of hair before showing scalp. Still, it was the beginning of a new state of mind brought about by the obvious – the classic bald-headedness that is the hallmark of the breast cancer patient. Deep breath, dear self. The hair will eventually grow back.

Unlike some proactive cancer patients, I did not want to help it along. There would be no head shaving for me. I wanted to hang on to that hair for a few more days, like a child trying to prolong the life of a rapidly melting ice cream cone on a hot summer day.

I didn't want to have to wear that wig to work for another week. It's funny, the arbitrary and fairly meaningless goalposts you set for yourself. I vowed to make it through one more workweek with my own hair, and decided to make a game out of it. I think that's the key. Whether you choose to shave your head or let your hair fall out in due course, do whatever works for you.

For the rest of the week I awoke with more strands of hair on my pillow and stuck to my face. My morning pre-work routine grew slightly longer as I determinedly arranged and sprayed my remaining strands into submission. The roots could let go during the day, but done up in a ponytail and plenty of hairspray, I could fake it for a couple more days. Such stubbornness. I had to laugh at my own ridiculous game. I suppose it was about having some measure of control over the uncontrollable. In any case, I had fun with it.

When Saturday arrived, I could fake it no longer. I was going bald, and rapidly. Jim, a barber in his younger years, cut the remaining long strands and I was left with a just a thin layer of short hair, hanging on ever so gingerly. He said I looked cute, but I didn't feel cute.

In the immortal words of *Seinfeld's* George Costanza, "These are the historic remains of a once great society of hair."

At the same time, my mouth began to heal and my revulsion to food was beginning to let up a bit. I still had a few days to enjoy the respite before my next chemo.

Since eating was once again a pleasurable experience, we decided to go out for lunch. I was no longer comfortable with my head. After a lifetime of thick hair, the breeze felt strange and I didn't like it. For the first time, I covered my head with a hat and wore it all the way through our meal. When we returned home, I switched to a kerchief, which was surprisingly comfortable. I'd turned a corner.

I turned another corner on Monday morning, when I showed up for work with a wig on top of my freshly smooth head. I felt as conspicuous as the day I first showed up using a walking cane a few years before. I hated drawing attention to myself, especially for health reasons, but I didn't want to hide, either. I purposely visited the most populated area of the building so everyone could get a good look at me all at once and we could move on. Approval all around. "Sophisticated...cute...pixie-like...cool..."

Me? "Pixie-like?" Well, what else could they say?

Liz would be arriving that evening, and it felt wrong, somehow, to greet her in the wig. I wouldn't be the Mom she was expecting. Well, I would, but I wouldn't look like her, and I wouldn't feel like her. I felt like an imposter in my own skin.

I saw it on her face the moment our eyes met and I instantly regretted the public surprise. I probably should have warned her. She saw the wig and was momentarily taken aback. Then she smiled as she saw beyond the wig and our history together blended with this new reality.

Her visit would last 15 days, but we couldn't wait to hunker down together and put on our virtual silly hats. That's what I miss most about not living near my children. The silly things.

With the effects of chemo wearing off and Liz's visit, it was time to take inventory. When you first learn you have cancer, you go into cancer mode. You have to learn all you can, make important decisions, choose doctors, and take the first steps toward eradicating it from your body. It is a necessary phase in which cancer must be the primary focus.

Once you're underway and doing what you believe must be done, it's time to get back to the business of living. You can't be all about cancer. You have to get back to doing things for the sheer joy of doing them. If you can't keep up with your former schedule, you can still find ways to enjoy yourself. You have to continue living or you're going to lose yourself.

The second round of chemo would soon be upon us, so we decided to begin her visit with a good old-fashioned pajama party like we used to enjoy when she and her brothers were little.

After dinner, we abandoned Jim (or gave him the night off, depending on how you look at it) and put on our coziest pajamas. Then we gathered up some pillows, blankets, and assorted snacks and headed to the downstairs family room. I was fighting extreme fatigue, but still determined to have a good time. I mean, really, how are you going to pass up an opportunity for some girl time?

It wasn't the first, and certainly wouldn't be the last time I would decide to set aside fatigue and other health problems in favor of a good time. The road of life is uncertain, filled with twists and turns we never see coming. What's around the next bend, or where the road finally ends, none of us can say. I'm just happy to be on the road at all, and as long as I am, I'm going to make the most of it.

We began work on a 1,500-piece jigsaw puzzle, turned on an inconsequential movie, and broke out the snacks. More than any of those activities, it was about girl talk. Unlike days of old, I could only nibble at the goodies and it took me four hours to drink one bottle of hard lemonade, which caused me to hiccup uncontrollably for several hours. That only made us laugh more, so determined were we to live in the moment. Our silliness alternated with heart-to-heart talks in which we shared our innermost feelings and shed more than a few tears. It was a real chick fest.

In the wee hours of the morning, we came around to what we both knew was unavoidable. There were only a few people who would want to, or that I would want to view my battle scars in their full glory. Liz, of course, was one of them. She wanted to, so off came the top for inspection. No more mystery. It brought us closer than ever.

It was 4:00 a.m. when I could fight sleep no longer and closed my eyes, drifting off with a smile on my face.

On the morning of my second round of chemo, Jim left for the doctor's office in our car, while Liz and I followed in mine. Jim wanted to be present when I met with our oncologist, but Liz wanted to stay for the chemo. Patients were allowed only one visitor at a time, so Jim gave up his spot to Liz. We all knew how difficult that was for him. In the end, it would be the only session he missed.

For this session, I was directed to a second chemo room upstairs. This overflow room was smaller and had a cozier feeling, but served as a reminder of the overwhelming number of cancer patients.

Round two went off pretty well, sparing my veins from multiple stabs. I accepted a warm blanket and settled in with my darling Liz by my side. She has a way of injecting humor into things and taking the edge off.

I tried to fight the drowsiness that came with the first fluids, but I faded in and out of sleep. Liz and I chatted as one bag was switched out for the next. Then I joined the bathroom parade. One after another, we patients would gather ourselves together, unplug various machines, and point our IV poles toward the bathroom. As soon as I would return to my recliner, I would feel the need to go again. Damn fluids. It reminded me of being pregnant. All in all, it was a smooth session, and it was fun having Liz with me.

For the next few days, she also accompanied me to work, hanging out in my office, which I think amused the rest of the staff. My office was small and narrow. Actually, I think it was a converted storage closet. It was one hundred times brighter with Liz in it.

During her visit, whenever Liz and I left the house, Jim asked her to take the wheel. They both felt that my reflexes were not up to the task. It was interesting to watch Liz and her stepfather exchange That Look while discussing what would be in my best interests. Even though they both treated me with the utmost respect, it felt as if Liz had stepped into a parental role. They were partners in watching out for me, and that was both comforting and unsettling.

While she was still in town, I put off my writing assignments so I could spend more time with her. Over the weekend, the three of us enjoyed a pleasant day in the cool, crisp sunshine of a local vineyard. We took several hours to slowly sip our wine and take in the splendid mountain views of the Shenandoah Valley. There's nothing quite like a mountain view to remind you how connected we are to the earth.

I say it a lot because it is the truth – the heart of life is in the simple things. If you've been too busy to notice that, please take the time to think about it and savor what's right in front of you.

CHAPTER 9

In the Thick of It

It would be an understatement to say that January passed in a blur. After all three of my children came and went, I felt a sudden void, a lack of anticipation of something beyond work and chemo and my struggle with food. There were no more family visits, no holidays, no special events scheduled in the near future. I ran out of non-cancer related things on which to focus.

Once my third round of chemo was administered, a thick fog settled in my brain. I did what was necessary. I got up each morning, went to work, came home and attacked my writing. Then I prepared dinner and settled in to read or watch television with Jim.

On weekends, we cleaned the house and ran errands. Occasionally, we took leisurely walks or went to the movies. We were living a seemingly routine life, not much different than the lives of everyone else on our street, our block, and our neighborhood.

As I went through these motions, it was difficult to hang on to a single train of thought for long. Sleep and wakefulness, dreams and reality all ran together in the mush that had taken the place of my brain. Despite all that, there was no sense of doom and gloom.

Back when my MS was in its heyday, the afternoon nap was a necessary event. MS-related fatigue was so strong that I often fell asleep while sitting up and working on my laptop. The new, cancer-related fatigue was different. It was fatigue that would not give in to sleep. I had no desire to nap. Taking to my bed, even for one day, was not an option I wanted to consider, my fear being that it would sap what little strength I had.

By the end of January, the writing that I so enjoyed was beginning to suffer. For me, one of the side effects of chemo was watery eyes, and I do mean watery. Mine were too watery to begin with, but the new tears were thick and sticky, causing blurred vision and the need to constantly dab at my face. Reading and writing were a struggle best left to small chunks of time.

I took to carrying around one of Jim's large white handkerchiefs so I could keep up with the unstoppable leak. Outside in the cold, my cheeks felt chapped from the moisture. To those who didn't know, I must have appeared to be the world's biggest sad sack. Maybe that's why strangers felt compelled to counsel me on positive attitude.

Meanwhile, my hatred of food raged on, having become a much bigger problem than I ever thought possible. In a purely evil twist, the healthy foods I so enjoyed, and which my body so desperately needed, became repulsive and almost impossible to eat. Even plain vegetables looked, smelled, and tasted like bitter poison. My favorite vegetable, the fresh, crisp green bean, became a vile sight on my dinner plate. Eating them became just another form of taking my medicine.

I had to keep reminding myself that for the time being, pleasure and eating were divorced. I had to focus on the fact that eating was about fueling a body under siege, so I willed myself to eat. As soon as I could, I'd brush my teeth in an attempt to erase all evidence of food.

Dr. G said these side effects usually occur much later in the chemo process and he was concerned about long-term problems, especially with cognitive function. I couldn't afford to lose any more weight and I was also becoming anemic.

During the three-week cycle, as soon as I would start to

feel relief, it was time to start all over again. As much as I disliked chemo, it never occurred to me that I could stop. No matter how awful I felt at any given time, I was determined not to lose sight of the aggressiveness of this particular cancer. I wanted to kick its ass but good. If it were to return, it would be much worse, and in my own mind, the first battle was winner take all.

The third chemo session started off badly. The nurse had tremendous difficulty getting the needle into my vein and keeping it there. That caused one of the larger veins to collapse and left an indentation that ran from the crook of my elbow to my wrist. After a few more painful attempts, another nurse succeeded in tapping into a suitable vein.

Several weeks later, my arm still hurt. Dr. G explained that the vein would never recover and my body would compensate by rerouting the blood flow through smaller veins. Since we only had one arm to work with anyway, he recommended that I have a chemo port installed under the skin of my chest. Following that, treatment could be administered through it rather than my arm.

The surgical outpatient procedure was fairly simple, I was told, but would require anesthesia. Two funny things happened at the hospital that morning. Even though I was as bald as a newborn baby, they insisted I wear a hair net for surgery. Rules are rules, I suppose. It was an interesting look, that's for sure.

Secondly, they gave me an information card for the chemo port, which I was to carry with me in case of emergency. The info came with a wristband which the nurse removed as she said, "Oh, you don't want to wear this…we stopped handing these out because they're the same color as the 'Do Not Resuscitate' wrist bands!" Alrighty, then…we don't want anyone to make that mistake.

I didn't know the surgeon who installed the port. He said it didn't matter which side he used, so I chose the side that was already messed up. A new bump and a new scar wouldn't make much of a difference. The port was inserted entirely under the skin, so there was no maintenance for me to perform. The nurses would flush it regularly and use it for blood work, as well as chemotherapy, by poking a needle through my skin. It would be a welcome relief to my poor, overworked left arm.

Of course, nothing is ever as simple as all that. Dr. M, my breast surgeon, was not at all happy with the placement of the device on my right side. She felt strongly that it should have been on the non-surgical side to avoid complications, especially since lymph nodes were removed. Her argument made sense, but it was decided that leaving it in would cause less potential for a problem than moving it. The chemo port would need to be surgically removed once treatment was completed.

My chest, at least on the right side, appeared to be nothing but skin and bones and a bump where the port was located. I was so unfamiliar with my new landscape I thought I'd discovered new lumps, which Dr. M politely, and with a straight face, informed me were my ribs. Oops. I hadn't seen those since I was a pre-teen. I wonder how she kept from laughing.

She also felt I was ready to order a prosthetic breast, one month ahead of schedule, because of my quick healing process. A doctor's prescription for a prosthetic breast and mastectomy bras meant that these costs could go toward my deductible.

After work the very next day, I went over to the medical supply store and tried on some new breasts, or I should say a new breast. Now if that isn't a weird experience, I don't know what is.

It wasn't like trying on a new pair of shoes, and not quite like trying on a wig. This thing was going to become an important part of my attire for the rest of my life.

Mastectomy bras come with pockets that keep the prosthesis close to the chest. The prosthesis itself has some weight to it, which helps it to stay in place, giving you a more balanced feeling.

I chose the skimpiest bras first, but quickly found out they couldn't cover everything I needed them to cover. Even though I'm small breasted, the difference between Pristine and the mastectomy side was far greater than you'd expect, and it takes one hell of a good bra make it work.

They told me I'd even be able to wear my prosthesis in the ocean or in a swimming pool without causing damage. That's another thing. I'd need to buy a mastectomy bathing suit to hold my prosthesis. Either that, or sew some pockets in them. Alas, all my bathing suits were cut in such a way as to make that unworkable.

It requires someone with experience to help you choose just the right prosthetic and bras. It was strange, to say the least, to bare my scarred chest to this stranger in a store and have her stand and stare, checking every angle and pulling and tugging at the bras. How odd, to watch someone hold your breast in the palm of her hand.

The prosthetic allowed me to wear some of my old clothes again, but certainly not all of them. These days, when I'm dressed, I feel as two-breasted as ever. It is only when I take off my bra that I'm reminded of what's missing. Even now, low necklines and loose-fitting tops that separate from the body when I bend forward are a no-no. Horizontal stripes and V-necks only help to accentuate my unevenness, but there are far worse things in life.

My first real bra with actual cups! It was cream colored and had a delicate pink bow between the cups. I struggled with the two little hooks in the back, and then straightened the straps. I studied my reflection in the mirror, standing straight and proud. Just like my big sister and my mother...I'm a woman now.

There's something about breasts that confounds me. How could these body parts come to mean so many things in our culture? Little girls can't wait to try on their first bra and teens can't wait to show off their cleavage. Healthy women with perfectly lovely breasts opt for surgery to enhance what nature gave them. And where would the advertising industry be without breasts? Breasts are big business, used in marketing everything from cars to beer. Music videos, movies, celebrities...you can't avoid breasts bouncing all over the place. And we have a lot of names for them, some that are quite demeaning. It's all part of our culture.

Ah, but unbutton your shirt to breastfeed your baby and it's a completely different story. *Wouldn't you be more comfortable in the restroom? Put those things away! Nobody wants to see that!* We really need to get to get a grip.

I never had much in the way of cleavage, but now I don't even have that. I'm a one-breasted wonder, but I'm still me. Breasts don't make the woman.

Up until I actually had that prosthesis and bra in hand, I hadn't touched my bra drawer or discarded my old bras. I held on to the ridiculous notion that I might need them someday, even though I knew I wouldn't. And maybe I'd sew pockets in them to create my own mastectomy bras. Nah, too skimpy and too little coverage. There was no saving them.

I pulled the drawer open and decided it was time to do the deed. Lacy bras, strapless bras, plunging bras, sapphire blue, midnight black, beige bras, and bras with matching panties. All the pretty little bras...thank you for your service, but it's time for you to go, time to put the past in the past and move forward. Into a bag they went, but it was not easy to discard them. It was so very final. I think at least one of the tears that slid down my cheek was the real deal.

Writing. Why did I ever think I could write, I wondered. I drafted *No More Secs!* and before I could do anything with it, I was diagnosed with cancer. The manuscript was languishing in the pile of unfinished work that was my life.

Jim was going to design the book cover, edit, code it for

Kindle and Nook, and take care of all the publication details, but he lost interest as other concerns wrestled to the surface.

In addition to helping me deal with cancer treatment, Jim managed to somehow maintain his own work schedule. Often, he could be found writing code and tweaking websites long after I settled into bed.

The stupid book was lingering proof of my own foolishness. A writer, indeed. Who was I kidding? It's amazing how quickly things can change.

But what if I didn't make it through the cancer? What if I died and my little book never saw the light of day? I wanted to see it published while I was still alive. The book had to happen, damn it. I asked Jim to help me make it happen. Suddenly it became of the utmost importance to me. Perhaps the new/old project was just what we needed.

The day-to-day details of life, making a living, hopes and dreams, exhausting cancer treatment, and trying to keep our heads above water was, to put it mildly, emotionally exhausting.

My state of mind was captured in this journal entry:

> "I don't mean to be a downer, but this is how I feel today...people are always commenting on how wonderfully I'm doing and how they admire my strength and attitude...and what can I say? I AM doing well, I DO have a good attitude, and I AM strong...but I can't keep that up 24/7.
> Sometimes I am simply sick and tired and drained and need to just let myself be that for a little while."

CHAPTER 10

Kissed By An Angel

Time continued to test me as days and nights blended together. From the funeral home to my writing desk to the dinner table and to bed, I did what I was supposed to do on automatic pilot. A haze of chemo and exhaustion and fighting the fight left me no energy or time to organize my own thoughts.

Despite family support, the geographical divide meant that we were very much on our own. Back in 2004, a doctor suggested I check out a local MS support group, so I attended a meeting. I immediately felt completely lost in the crowd. I wasn't comfortable with it, didn't feel the need for it, and never went back.

I knew there was a breast cancer support group in town, but I didn't have the energy or the inclination to look into it. I read about breast cancer patients who went for massages, meditation, acupuncture, or yoga. Some took up tai chi, went on retreats, or had spa days. There's good in that, I know, but I had too much on my plate to give it much consideration. Where they found the time, the energy, and the budget to do those things while going through cancer treatment was beyond me, anyway.

My therapy was in my routine. It came in the form of long, leisurely walks and phone chats with my children. It was in hanging around with Jim, taking in a Sunday afternoon movie, or playing a game.

I found therapy in my writing, and in the quest to see my book make it into the hands of readers. It was in life itself.

Despite my physical discomfort and the uncertainty of my future, I was grateful for each day that I could enjoy these simple pleasures. My therapy was in not having the time or desire for sick days.

For some people, therapy might come in the form of mountain climbing or white water rafting. It might mean staying in five-star hotels and dining in world-class restaurants. Maybe it means a weekend on a beach. Whatever living means to you – that's what you need to hold on to when your life is at stake. Don't let anyone else tell you what you should or should not be doing.

I only had to get through one more chemotherapy session before we switched to a new regimen. I looked forward to the change, because with each change I was advancing closer to the finish line.

When we arrived for the fourth and final chemo of phase one, my blood work left much to be desired, and we were sent home without treatment. As Dr. G put it, "I'm trying to kill cancer cells, I'm not trying to kill you."

That was, in a weird way, extremely disappointing. Even a minor delay made the whole process seem as though it would never conclude. Happily, the one-week reprieve did give me back myself, if only briefly.

Finally, the fourth session was completed. Naturally, all the old side effects came along with it, but onward and upward...

One week later, we would begin the second phase of chemotherapy. Twelve weeks to go. As I crossed that threshold, the last remnants of my eyelashes disappeared and my eyebrows were getting rather sparse. Make-up was unable to mask my pallor and, if I didn't apply it correctly, only brought more attention to my frailties.

Anemia, not an uncommon side effect of chemo, was getting a little worse with each treatment, and was probably the reason for my ongoing fatigue. It wasn't bad enough to require treatment at that point, but definitely something we had to keep an eye on. Dr. G spoke of the potential for long-term health consequences, but it was his hope, and ours, that those things would not come to pass. Careful monitoring would suffice for the time being.

For the first time since we began seeing him, Dr. G hugged me on my departure, saying he admired my spirit. I'm not sure what I said to prompt that response, but it felt good. Doctors take note: a show of compassion is good medicine. I'm sure some patients have no desire to be hugged by a doctor, but a simple acknowledgement of the situation, from one person to another, can go a long way.

Dr. G, Dr. M, and their respective practices, gave me a new enthusiasm for the medical profession. Maybe it's cancer that makes a difference. I'll never know for sure, but I am very grateful to have happened upon their services.

The new chemo drug, Taxotere, came with a dose of steroids. I still had the sleepiness of the first wave of drugs as they pushed through my port, followed by a bit of a buzz, sort of like I get from a glass of wine. I rather enjoyed that part.

Then came restless legs...a real thing after all. I shall never scoff at restless leg syndrome again – it's a real bitch, I assure you. On day two, the steroids would cause an abundance of energy – and an unfortunate inability to sleep for more than a catnap, with a crash coming just before it was time for the next round. I became a night wanderer, searching for something to occupy my mind in the wee hours.

For the most part, I managed to maintain a weary, yet positive hold on life. Life was all about the cancer, but not about the cancer at all. It was about nothing and everything. We didn't dwell on it, or even speak of it much, but it was with us always.

More than anything, I wanted Jim to know that I wasn't all about me. As impossible as it was to escape cancer's grip at that point, he was on my mind always. I didn't want to lose the give and take of our relationship. I wanted to carry my own weight so he could catch a break.

Sadly, during 10 months of treatment, shockingly few people checked in to see how Jim was coping or to ask if he needed a hand. His strong presence and confident air apparently led people to believe that nothing had changed for him.

Please indulge me in a few words of advice. Most people won't take you up on a blanket statement like, "Let me know if you need anything." If you truly want to help, make a specific offer to do something tangible like running an errand, babysitting, cooking, cleaning, etc.

If you ever find yourself at a loss for what to do for a sick friend, try a phone call, a hug, a joke, or a smile. And don't forget spouses, children, or caregivers. They face different challenges, but they are challenges nonetheless.

It doesn't matter how far away you are – you can at least make that phone call. Not every illness is over and done with in a couple of weeks, so don't forget about your friend after the initial shock or after the first few months of treatment. Sometimes it's a very long haul, so let them know you're still a friend, no matter where the road leads or how long it takes to get there.

One day, an express package in the mailbox turned out to be a box of homemade cookies, sent by a faraway acquaintance. Cookies. Beautiful, tasty, cookies! How weird and wonderful that they actually tasted as cookies should taste and that I could enjoy eating a few! The enclosed note revealed that the sender thought the gesture was "kinda lame," but she wanted to let us know that she was thinking of us.

Lame? Absolutely not! Those are exactly the gestures that meant so much to me and to Jim. That's what makes life grand and that's the kind of thing I knew, immediately, that I must pay forward. I'll say it again: However awkward or difficult, however "lame" you fear your offering, just do it! Behold the power of the cookie.

Word was that my family members in Rhode Island were

organizing an 80th birthday party for Mom at the end of March. When I first heard about it, it was inconceivable to me that we could attend. Driving from Virginia to Rhode Island between chemo sessions seemed about as reasonable as shuttling out to the space station. Even if I felt up to it and if Jim didn't mind the drive, that would mean more work days lost and more additional expenses to absorb. That's hard to explain to people. Then again, I had cancer and my mother was turning 80. How many more opportunities would we have to be together?

I was already concerned about getting out to Illinois for Liz's college graduation in May. More than at any time in my life, I wanted to use my time wisely, to spend it with the people I love. But life doesn't always work out that way, does it?

The food wars took another prisoner. Popcorn. Everybody who knows me knows how much I love popcorn. Suddenly I couldn't stand it. Not the sight of it; not the smell of it. It seemed to me that a mouthful of Styrofoam would taste better and be easier to swallow. All those trips, fingers to bowl, all that chewing...what a lot of work for such an awful taste. It was exhausting just thinking about it. I hated the stuff and wondered if that would change after chemo. Then again, since I hated it anyway, what would it matter?

One day, I returned from my morning at work, completed an article that was due, and forced myself to get dinner on the table, though it was a strain. Sensing my subdued outlook, Jim brought up Mom's birthday party. He knew how important it was to me, and how disappointed I'd be if I missed it. As much as I wanted to go, the physical process of doing so was overwhelming to me. It couldn't be done, I insisted.

By 10:00 p.m. I was ready for sleep. A tickle in the back of my throat caused a coughing fit, rousing me from slumber. Jim brought me a glass of water and I was stunned to realize it was only 11:15 p.m. I would have sworn it was morning already. I continued to fade into and out of sleep, wet with perspiration and tired from tossing and turning. By 2:15 a.m. I could take it no longer and headed for the comfort of the sofa and the distraction of my laptop.

That about sums up most of my nights during chemotherapy. It was a black hole that knew nothing of time.

My cancer journal was something I started in October, shortly after diagnosis. I wanted to have a set of notes that contained dates, information about doctors and medications and the details of my medical care. It was intended to help me track important information and to help with health insurance paperwork, if necessary. That turned out to be very useful. Even now, it brings back some of the details that might otherwise have faded from memory.

Before I knew it, I was adding brief snippets about how I was feeling, both physically and emotionally. It was the writer in me, I guess. Once I started chemotherapy, finding the time and strength to make entries grew increasingly difficult. There are huge gaps in time followed by attempts to fill in the blanks in one fell swoop.

An entry from March reflects the foggy state of being in which I lived:

> "I've been kissed by an angel...not literally, but that's what I'm calling it. While taking a break from cleaning yesterday, I found myself in a half-awake half-asleep state and I felt a soft kiss in the middle of my forehead. Jim was not in the room. I couldn't identify the kiss as coming from a male or female, child or adult, but it was pleasant and made me smile, in spite of the fact that I knew it to be a figment of my imagination.

> "A few hours later, I took another catnap and the same thing happened. Again, I was filled with a sense of peace and happiness.

> "During the night, while in a full sleep, I dreamed

about a white light, or possibly a white liquid, that touched the center of my forehead in the very same spot where the kisses landed. I knew it was a dream but, again, was filled with a peaceful feeling.

"I'm not one to claim I know what's going on beyond this life. I don't need to understand what it was, because even if it was nothing more than my own imagination, it was a positive feeling, one that I can conjure up again and again...a sort of meditation...and I am filled with a sense of peace. Whatever it was, it was a gift that I shall use again and again, and I'm calling it 'kissed by an angel.'"

Some people who go through chemo speak of chemo smell. They describe a chemical odor that seems to flow from their pores. If I had that smell, I was unaware of it. There was a smell I associated with chemotherapy, though. The aroma came from a Subway shop, which was located upstairs from my doctor's office suite. Before I started chemo, it was a rather tempting smell, but soon became so associated with chemo that I could not imagine one without the other. To this day, I can't pass a Subway without a chemotherapy flashback.

When we arrived for my next session, Dr. G's office was jam-packed. So many people with cancer, and so many looking ill. We entered the treatment room when prompted, seeking my assigned nurse for the day, but there weren't any chemo chairs available. We had to sit off to the side to wait for my blood test.

As the nurse flushed my chemo port, I noticed a woman sitting diagonally from us. She had a blood pressure cuff on her ankle. Double mastectomy, I knew. Across the room, a woman wore a long sleeve on one arm. A lymphedema sleeve.

A few recliners over, a very frail-looking man sat quiet and still as a nurse attempted again and again to find a vein while his wife looked on, a pained expression on her face. It turned out to be his third bout with cancer, and his veins were uncooperative.

The chemotherapy room often buzzed with chatter and laughter, but sometimes the sights and sounds were stark reminders of the ongoing wars within its walls.

While she worked, Nurse Patty gave me a few tips on how to get around some of my more recent side effects. She's the kind of nurse who makes the going a little less rough.

Unfortunately, the results of my blood test were poor once again. Both my red and white blood counts were below the minimum acceptable levels to begin treatment, so Dr. G had to be consulted. Word came back that I would not receive chemotherapy that day, and an appointment was set for one week later. Even our best-laid plans, I reminded myself, were subject to change.

Patty assured us that it was not an uncommon event during chemo and that a week off would probably set things right again. She told us to watch for signs of infection, fever, or any illness, and to call immediately if I felt ill.

All things considered, we found it amazing that I continued to function so well. This body of mine does not quit easily. As much as I wanted to go home that day, I was deflated. I wanted to attack those cancer cells, not give them time to regroup. I didn't want to extend the process. That much longer to feel ill, that much longer to be hairless, that much longer until I could even think of uttering the words, "I am cancer-free."

Blood was showing up in tissues whenever I blew my nose. It's a common side effect of chemo and had been going on for a couple of weeks. Just a few days after the thwarted chemo session, blood began to intermittently drip out of my nose as I sat at my desk. I figured that was worth a phone call and soon I was back in the doctor's office for more blood work. This time they wanted to check my platelets. Following my usual course of not borrowing trouble, I didn't bother to ask what would happen if the blood tests didn't go well. Fortunately, it was a false alarm. The nurse said the chemo was probably affecting the membranes in my nose.

By the next Tuesday, my blood counts reached acceptable levels and it was game on again. Dr. G adjusted the medication, as well as the amount of steroids it contained, hoping to decrease the monstrous side effects. He said there is often a period of adjustment with dosage and the changes should not affect the overall effectiveness of treatment.

What a session it was. Rather than fading into and out of sleepiness as I usually did, I fell stone cold asleep! I'd been watching others sleep through it for months. Some even snored right through it. Oh, I didn't want to be a public snorer!

During a half-awake/half-asleep delusion of sorts, I began to speak nonsense to Jim. I heard myself talking and knew full well that I was not making the slightest bit of sense, but I kept jabbering anyway, as uncontrolled as a runaway train. Before chemo was over that day, the foggy feeling cleared up and I felt compelled to explain to Jim that I knew I was talking nonsense when I was doing it and since I was aware of it, I couldn't be crazy. Huh? The more I tried to explain, the more I sounded like a drunk pretending to be sober, and you know how that usually works out. Thankfully, it was an isolated episode.

A series of delays caused our session to take up most of the day. I did feel a bit guilty that I managed to get some good shut-eye while Jim had to stay awake through the whole ordeal.

Beyond the doors of the chemo room exists an army of mystery elves, anonymous people who donate handmade hats and blankets to chemotherapy patients. Some bring goodies like hard candies to share with those who can't stomach food. These little treasures mean so much to the people receiving treatment.

A handmade blue crocheted shawl/blanket got me through some chemo sessions and will always serve as a reminder –

not of chemo, but of the spirit of giving. Too bad the givers aren't always around to see the recipient's smile, but I guess deep down inside they know. My deep appreciation goes out to the person who created my little blanket. You did good.

CHAPTER 11

Wings

Early on, one of my editors asked if I was interested in writing about my cancer ordeal, but I couldn't wrap my chemo fog head around the concept. By the middle of March, the time felt right.

If I was overly concerned about privacy, certainly publishing a memoir about MS wasn't the way to go. Still, it's difficult to write about something so monumental and personal when you don't have any clue how it's all going to turn out. It seemed like a good idea to share the story of an average person with MS who suddenly found herself battling cancer.

I submitted the first post in a series, hoping my story might serve as a timely reminder for women to perform breast self-exams and not to ignore breast lumps. For the most part, that's what happened, but as I continued the series, there was a disturbing element for which I was unprepared. Since I had limited energy, I was unable to respond to it properly.

They'd show up in the comments section, but mostly they'd email me directly. "You have no clue," one wrote. "You're sending a very dangerous message."

I was taken to task for having a mastectomy – a procedure nothing short of mutilation, according to them. There's never a good reason for a mastectomy. It's the coward's way out. The medical establishment wants to kill you...a biopsy will only spread the cancer...the cure for cancer is (take your pick) a raw diet, vitamin supplements, marijuana, yoga, positive attitude, God, meditation, imagery, bravery, chanting, etc. You name it; it's a cure, and each writer is 100 percent certain of it. Too bad they can't agree on what that cure is.

There was no shortage of theories on why people get cancer, either. It might be because you're a bad person (tell that to the parent of a sick child), or maybe you're paying for your sins from a previous life. Karma. It might be because you think about cancer and try to avoid it and thereby invite it in. You didn't learn the secret of life. It may be because you saw a doctor in the first place – doctors give you cancer, you know.

One woman wrote me repeatedly, intent on shoving her own theory down my throat. She claimed to have had and beaten breast cancer without the help of modern medicine. Found the lump herself, she did, but she wasn't foolish enough to see a doctor or get one of those killer biopsies. No ma'am, not her. Just decided right then and there to cure her self-diagnosed cancer using a raw vegan diet, and guess what? It worked! Self-diagnosed, self-treated, self-cured, self-righteous, and from my perspective, quite delusional.

One man accused me of being an alarmist, writing that you should try fixing your diet before running off to see a doctor.

Make no mistake about it – I'm all for a healthy diet. In fact, I strongly encourage you to learn more about the foods you eat and how they impact your health. It's something we should all be doing throughout our lives, not just when we get sick. Food is how we fuel our bodies and we should not take that responsibility lightly. The same goes for products we use on our bodies or around our homes. However, I stand by my advice to see a doctor right away when you find a lump in your breast.

It was emotionally exhausting. What began as a hopeful message slowly turned into a negative. I was disheartened and discouraged, and it was reflected in future posts. I lost my focus.

Now, if I knew for sure exactly what causes or cures cancer, or MS for that matter, I'd be shouting it from the mountaintops. What I do know is that if your cancer or MS is self-diagnosed, I'm not interested in your cure. I also know that wishing cancer away will not make it so. While the choices I made were unpleasant, they were informed choices based on the particulars of my medical history and advice from qualified professionals who actually examined me and studied my test results.

I don't offer medical advice because I am not qualified to do so. However, I do recommend seeking medical attention if you believe you have a life-threatening illness. It doesn't mean you have to take the advice of your doctor. It doesn't mean you have to take the same road I took or even that it's necessary. It doesn't mean you can't pursue alternative or complementary treatment. It does mean that you'll get more information on which to base those decisions. You can still change bad dietary habits or quit smoking or make any other lifestyle adjustments that will help improve your overall health.

I also recommend that you not compare your situation to anyone else's. If time is of the essence, burying your head in the sand could kill you. Consider that choices you make today may affect your quality of life tomorrow. Treat your body like the most important possession you have – because it is.

Another poor blood test caused my doctor to cancel chemo again, and again, I felt both relief and distress. It also resulted in an easing of side effects. Just a few days before the party, we made a spur of the moment decision to make the trek to Rhode Island, after all. What was I thinking, anyway? Life is for the living and I was still very much alive. How could I even consider not celebrating my mother's 80th birthday with her in person? It would fit in neatly between chemo sessions.

It would be a whirlwind two-day visit sandwiched in between two driving days. Jim does all the driving whenever we're on a road trip. It's a holdover from the days when MS made it difficult to move my legs or to hold my hands on the steering wheel for too long.

As is our custom, we spent most of our time on the road chatting and singing with the radio, my energy level buoyed by anticipation and a week free of chemo.

As we passed cities and towns along the way, I thought about the people who lived there. Undoubtedly, we passed more cancer wards and chemotherapy rooms, oncologists, surgeons, and nurses, and cancer patients, ever more cancer patients. I was not alone in this thing, I reminded myself. There could be no room for self-pity. Not ever.

I'm a people watcher. I like to pick people out of a crowd and imagine their story. What brought them to this place on this day? Where have they been and where are they going? I especially like to pick out that person who appears grouchy or moody and wonder what preceded that mood.

If there's one thing I know for certain in this life, it's that what we see with our eyes or hear with our ears is often misleading. I pay attention to my first impressions and listen to my gut instincts, but I'm not always right. I can change my opinion as the bigger picture emerges.

I have the kind of face that is easily misread. On more than one occasion, I accidentally turned on my laptop camera and nearly frightened myself to death. Why do I look so angry when I don't feel angry? I try to remedy that by making it a point to smile, but that ends up making me look half-crazed or delusional.

Those thoughts were weaving through my brain as we closed in on Rhode Island. I didn't want my constant tearing to blend in with my incorrect facial expressions and give the impression that I was a blubbering, angry mess. Then again, if anyone could read my face right, it would be my family. At least that's what I hoped.

I hadn't seen my younger brother in years. He and his

family were traveling in from Texas and I was very excited to visit with them. Oh, how comforting it was to be with the family again. My mother was at her finest, smiling and enjoying the celebration in her honor.

On our first night in town, she pulled me aside and asked if she could see my chest and bald head. We snuck away to a bedroom and closed the door. I removed my wig first. "I always thought I had a big head," I said, "but it's ridiculously tiny. I guess it was all hair!"

She laughed and rubbed my head. "You always did have a cute little head. And it's still cute."

I pulled my top over my head and took off my bra, fake breast and all. "Oh, that doesn't look too bad," she said. I showed her how the bra had pockets, pulled the prosthetic out, and placed it in her hand. She transferred it from one hand to the other, marveling at its weight and how the pocketed bra held it in place against my flesh. As I put myself back together she said, "You look perfectly natural. No one would ever guess."

Her matter-of-fact, but caring attitude struck just the right balance. I wasn't interested in being fawned over or draped in attention. I just wanted the feeling of family.

We all traipsed out to dinner and I got so caught up in the moment that I ordered a big plate of pasta primavera in olive oil and garlic. Surprisingly, I made quite a dent in it, too. None present could have imagined my struggles with food or fatigue. It's not that I could have planned it that way, but we were spared my post-chemo illness.

Later it was presents and cake and laughter and dozens of family photos, during which I was just Ann. Not Ann the cancer patient, but Ann the daughter, Ann the sister, Ann the aunt, Ann the wife. People who have cancer are just people, after all.

We posed again and again in groups large and small. Now the siblings; now the cousins; now the whole gang. On the sofa, standing, and in candid shots. We don't get together often, and it was an occasion we all wanted to remember.

We were barely settled in before it was time to hit the road again. Four hundred and eighty-five miles later, we flopped into our own bed, ready for a new dosage of poison to enter my body. No rest for the weary.

Back in the chemo chair, I noticed a younger-looking woman seated in a recliner across from me. I never saw her before, but we overheard her say that she had triple-negative breast cancer. That was enough for us to strike up a conversation with her.

The 31-year-old mother of two young girls had been in the process of preparing for reconstructive surgery following a double mastectomy. She was also considering having her ovaries removed when the cancer reappeared. It had metastasized to her liver and a few other organs. She was part of a clinical trial and said she was feeling well and optimistic about the future.

She was so thin, sitting in the big recliner with no one by her side. Her smile and her words told a tale of optimism, but her eyes reflected her struggle and much deeper concerns. Concerns, I'm sure, about her children, her husband, and her own life. I was deeply moved by this woman I would never cross paths with again. Hers is the face I see when I think about the reality of breast cancer. It's about babies losing their mothers, husbands losing their wives, parents losing their daughters. It's about a young woman's smile in the face of life and death struggle.

My heart went out to her and to her family. I was fortunate in so many ways. It was my first taste of survivor's guilt. She was so young and had such a young family. I had 51 years under my belt and my children were grown. Intellectually, I knew that guilt is a useless emotion in this situation and fairness has nothing to do with cancer. Emotionally, I felt as though some of my years should be turned over to her.

During those months of weekly chemotherapy sessions, I managed to continue working at the funeral home, minus one morning a week for chemo. Things were shifting at work, particularly for my job. As we turned the corner into April, I decided not to shift with them. It really wasn't about the cancer, it was just time to move on. With everything we were dealing with, the funeral home was no longer a good fit for us. After eight years on a job I only expected to have for a short while, life was taking me in a new direction.

You might think I took that leap because I wanted to rest and regroup, but nothing could be further from the truth. I viewed that change as an opportunity to dive headlong into the life of a freelance writer. Given the times, it was a strange, some might say unwise, decision. Making a living as a writer, particularly on a freelance basis, is a common dream, but not a practical one. Muddy waters, at best, but as long as life was making us juggle, why not throw another ball into the air?

My first order of business would be to remind Jim, now on a daily basis, that we needed to get *No More Secs!* to market. Secondly, I sought out and snagged a few new writing ventures.

Can you imagine two people spending virtually all their time together? We began our workday just a few feet from the bedroom, sitting at our matching desks, each lost in our own projects. I quickly fell into a groove and did my best to keep up.

The freelance life requires great discipline. Most people think the hardest part is to ignore potential distractions and remain focused on the job. For Jim and me, the hard part is tearing ourselves away from our work. That's bound to happen when you make a career out of something you enjoy.

I made it a policy to always dress before entering the office. No pajamas, no robes, no sweats. I also made it a policy not to ever bring my laptop or work-related papers into the bedroom. Jim and I wanted some clear dividing lines between our work and non-work worlds. I must admit to bringing the laptop into the kitchen while I prepare meals, though. You can do a lot of writing while dinner is simmering on the stove. I get some of my best ideas in the kitchen.

On sunny days, I'd grab my trusty MacBook and work at the bistro table on our deck, surrounded by pine trees and birds and sunshine. How I would make this new career path work was a mystery to me, but I've spent most of my life flying by the seat of my pants. It was probably a good sign that I still had wings.

CHAPTER 12

Go Toward the Light

Several chemo sessions in a row without a break caused side effects to mount. Exhausted, I hit the sheets early one night, intent on escape through sleep. Glorious, deep sleep was easy to achieve, but it didn't last.

As I shifted my position, my left eyelid opened just enough to see one pinpoint of super bright light shining straight into my field of vision. It came from nowhere in particular, and penetrated my eyes. It was so white that it was blinding.

Was I supposed to "go toward the light?" Was I dead?

Ever since I started chemo, I had this feeling that I might just shrink and fade away into oblivion. I actually felt as though my physical self could simply disappear. Maybe it was really happening.

If I am dead – and still conscious – it's a very encouraging sign, that's for sure. I wondered if I should remain still or try to move; should I feel excited or wary?

I blinked my eyes hard several times in an effort to clear my vision and take in my surroundings. The bright light was coming from the mirrored closet door and I could see Jim sitting up in bed. What's he doing in there? I reached for my eyeglasses and soon my world was clear once more. Jim was reading his Kindle...while using a small light...causing a reflection in the mirror...to shine into my face.

That's what happens when you're nearsighted and half asleep. You think you've seen the light.

That wasn't the last of my chemo-brain-induced visions. A few nights later, I dreamed that I was floating above our bed, not above my own body, as you might expect, but above Jim's, which I thought was weird. I was as light as air, happy, and looking down on him. His breathing was steady and he was sleeping peacefully, unaware of my ghostly presence. My heart was filled with love.

Blackness surrounded me. Not negative blackness; it was more like nighttime fog or smoke, wrapping around me like a gentle hug. I felt that if I wanted to, I could float clear through the ceiling, above the roof, and out into the wide open spaces.

As wonderful as it felt, I didn't want to stray any further from Jim. I knew – with absolute certainty – that if I floated beyond the ceiling of our bedroom, I'd be unable to return. Ever. I didn't want to leave him that way. I couldn't leave him alone just yet. I wasn't ready to go and I had to find a way to push myself back down.

Then I woke up in my usual place in bed beside him.

You don't have to be a psychiatrist to figure out why I had these strange thoughts and dreams. All I can say is that they were powerful and probably helped me to cope with whatever fears I held at bay during my waking hours. On those nights when I have trouble falling asleep, I can still conjure up that floating on air feeling.

Back in the food wars, the metal taste finally left me, but it was replaced by something far worse. My mouth began to feel like a sugar-laden disaster and my taste buds became wildly out-of-whack. The only foods that tasted right were sweets, and that's not at all what my body needed. I also had some luck with very spicy foods. Everything else, from soup to nuts, either had no taste at all or tasted like someone poured buckets of sugar over it. It was a sickeningly sweet taste that no one could explain and that I could not shake.

Oh, I how I came to miss the taste of a garden salad

tossed with olive oil and red wine vinegar, Brussels sprouts with garlic, and the aroma of black coffee in the morning. It's very strange to put a food you always enjoyed in your mouth and find it completely unappealing. Little things help to make up the whole of who we are and what we know about ourselves. When you lose those little things, it's like being a toddler and learning all about yourself again.

My favorite time of day was when I stood at the kitchen sink, doing the dinner dishes. It meant I didn't have to eat anymore and could dismiss all thoughts of force-feeding myself for the day.

So here's the part where things get unpleasant, but you really don't want to read a day-by-day account of those side effects any more than I want to write about them. They're boring and tedious.

It's amazing how quickly people can adjust to new physical realities, and how we can continue to function and even thrive while these things rage on. There comes a day when you realize that life is too precious to waste on the small stuff, and you begin to shift more and more items into that small stuff category. In fact, most things eventually end up there. As long as you're alive, you might as well concentrate on the good stuff.

The flip side of that is that I don't want sugarcoat cancer or cancer treatment. Don't let anybody kid you – chemotherapy is not easy and when it lasts more than six months, the side effects do pile on. Trust me on that. When you encounter someone going through extended chemotherapy, assume that for every visible side effect you see, like a bald head, there are a dozen side effects you don't see.

I'll spare us all and shorthand the whole thing into one paragraph. From the beginning of December until the end of June, I experienced loss of all body hair, excessive tearing from both eyes, bloody gums, mouth sores, sore teeth, sore throat, dry mouth, bloody nose, difficulty breathing due to blood in my nose, metal taste in my mouth, sickeningly sweet taste in my mouth, nausea, food revulsion, loss of appetite, weight loss, fatigue, sleep disturbances, nightmares, brittle and yellowed fingernails and toenails, constipation, bloody stools, anemia, difficulty concentrating, slowed reflexes, swollen feet, and chemo fog.

At least those are the things I can recall now. I didn't have every symptom every day, of course, but they became a constant throughout the process, something that just became part of daily life. You can let them take over your every waking thought or you can deal with them as you go. You wake up in the morning, do what you can to cope with the day's symptoms, and move on, because this is another day of life and you can take it or leave it.

There were days where my body felt so small, so diminished and disconnected from my spirit, that it could at any moment be carried away with the lightest breeze.

That's why you should never assume that just because someone is showing up at work and smiling that everything is coming up roses. Humor is great, but it's not enough. Cut them some slack; ask how they're doing; offer an empathetic ear; hand them a covered dish to take home. That's all it takes to make a difference.

For whatever reason, Jim and I were able to work around these temporary inconveniences. Living with MS probably helped prepare us for cancer treatment. If you're going to continue living – I mean really living through a major health crisis – you have to be flexible. You must be able to change your plans on a dime rather than allow troubles to sideline you.

Now that we've moved beyond treatment, I don't give those side effects much thought, except when my senses trigger a memory and I have an "oh, yeah..." moment.

Anytime we want to spend a holiday with family, it means we must travel. That's just the way it is. Fortunately, we enjoy traveling together by car. We often spend Easter with

Jim's family in New Jersey, so we didn't see any reason not to. Did I feel or look my best? Absolutely not. We did have a good time in the car, listening to a book on tape, at least when I wasn't nodding off to sleep.

The sights and smells of food preparation lasted most of the day and, at times, were almost too much to bear. I longed to be anywhere where food was not. But I acted as though I felt well; I ate as though hungry; and held my head high as though I was the most vibrant woman on earth. That's where the "fake it 'til you make it" mentality kicks in. As you socialize, you begin to leave your troubles for another day. It's a philosophy that works for me.

My next chemo session was scheduled for Tuesday, so we set out for home on Monday. The quick trip was, however, fairly exhausting, and I was thrilled to return home and to my normal routine.

Jim was taking on the lion's share of chores, both indoors and out, but I managed enough so that I felt I was doing my share, considering the circumstances. That's how marriage is supposed to work. All things may be equal, but they don't have to be equal all the time. They can tilt one way or the other when circumstances warrant it.

Creating simple goals for myself was something I started years before, when MS was having its way with me. Back then, I declared that no matter what – no matter how weak I felt – that I would always plan my activities so that I had enough strength to prepare dinner.

Having cancer was no reason to change that goal. Not that I made gourmet meals. When the situation called for it, I took every shortcut I could, and we did sometimes venture out for dinner.

Work and treatment and maintaining our home and property took all our time and attention. There was little opportunity, not to mention energy, for socializing. While our far-off friends and family were supportive, in some respects, Jim and I lived on a secluded island, alone in our daily struggle. I suspect it is that way for a lot of other people, too. We performed our dance on a high wire while juggling sharp objects, but we did it together. We didn't fall and we didn't get cut.

A few weeks later, another chemo session was cancelled due to poor blood work. Dr. G wanted me to regain some strength before assaulting my body again. With only six sessions to go, I was getting very excited about nearing the end.

The season of road trips continued, as there was another very important one that I simply would not consider cancelling. Liz would be graduating from Southern Illinois University at Carbondale in May, and I was determined to celebrate it with her in person. David and Tommy would be in town, too, so it was the perfect opportunity to see them all at once.

Jim made hotel reservations, got the car in shape, and arranged for our neighbors to check in on Smokey during our absence. All I had to do was keep myself together.

The kids hadn't seen me in person for months, and I knew my physical appearance would be startling, but I wanted them to see that I was stronger than I seemed. I chose my clothes carefully, trying not to appear lost in them.

Liz took us around campus and we walked the winding trails in the crisp spring air, delighting in the sights and sounds of college life. So much promise!

The graduation ceremony went off without a hitch. Liz was radiant and we were all so proud of her and her plan to attend graduate school. We only had a few days to spend together and we stuck with simplicity. We sat around Liz's apartment. We talked, joked, held hands, and played Wii.

After David and Tommy set off for home, Jim and I took Liz out for ice cream. I decided to take a wig break and tied a colorful scarf around my head. I didn't wear scarfs in public often because it seemed on par with wearing a sandwich board sign that says, "I have cancer." On the other hand, it was a lot comfier than the wig and more colorful than my hat. I wasn't comfortable, even around my home, with nothing on my bald head. It was way too breezy up there.

Jim opened the back of the Subaru so we could sit while we enjoyed ice cream cones. As we stood at the order window, I realized that the thought of ice cream was fun in spirit, but that I didn't really want to eat it. I sipped a cup of water while Jim and Liz worked on their cones. My sunglasses helped shield my sensitive eyes from the sun, but the trail of tears that became my constant companion could not be stopped. A slight breeze felt just right on my skin.

I never learned how to tie a head scarf correctly. I never learned how to do any of those traditionally girly things correctly. I've always admired women who know how to drape themselves in scarves and pashminas, layer their clothes just right, and carry off big, bold jewelry. I never could make so much as a ponytail without a mirror and a half dozen aborted attempts. I have the best of intentions, but I always end up looking like a little girl playing dress up with Mommy's clothes.

The breeze worked on the scarf until it became undone and slid off my slippery head. Try as I might, I couldn't manage to get it tied up just right. I could be wrong, but I think Jim and Liz were having a little laugh watching me attempt to make it work. I only ended up with an oversized knot, a lopsided scarf, and beads of perspiration dripping down my temples. I decided that from that point on, I'd stick with hats.

We took two days for the drive back home, which always seems so much longer than the drive out. This time, I gave in to the fatigue and let myself fade into and out of slumber without a fight.

Once we returned home, there were no more trips on the horizon, no more visits, and nothing in particular to plan. We would fall into our routine once and focus on getting through treatment.

Seeing the kids again gave me peace of mind. I saw that they were strong of body and of spirit. Good people. Independent, intelligent, and kind. They're young, but they, too, recognize and appreciate the simple joys of life. There is no better medicine in the world.

CHAPTER 13

A Bend in the Road

When you begin chemotherapy, a lot of suggestions come your way. One constant seems to be makeup and makeovers. I get it, at least to a certain extent. I certainly wanted to look my best, and my morning routine didn't change much during treatment. I still applied some makeup and did what I could to maintain a pleasant appearance.

I once had a nice set of full, dark eyebrows and enjoyed the look that mascara gave to my ample eyelashes. I missed them, but after a few failed attempts at eye shadow and eyeliner, I decided to learn to live with it. The river flowing from my eyes didn't always flow straight down. Sometimes, the amount of liquid was so great that it squirted upward when I blinked, making eye makeup smear and streak. I'd rather have naked eyes than look like I'm testing my Halloween costume.

There was no way I was going to attempt to glue on eyelashes and take the chance of glue ending up in my eye or to have the lashes slide down my cheek. I never tried false eyelashes before and didn't see any scenario where I could make them work in the constant flow of tears. And fake eyebrows? That wasn't going to happen. I could just picture myself smiling at someone while an eyebrow drooped out of place. I would live in fear of looking like I had a caterpillar crawling up the side of my face.

I'm sure many women benefit from such things, but it wasn't for me. I stuck with the basics and left my eyes to their nakedness. The new me – take me or leave me. As long as I didn't have blood leaking from my nose and gums, I figured I was looking pretty good.

With only a few more chemotherapy sessions to go, we began discussions about radiation and follow up care with Dr. G. His philosophy was very much in line with our own. Jim and I did not intend to spend our days on the patient merry-go-round or running in fear of a cancer recurrence.

Triple-negative breast cancer has a higher rate of recurrence than other breast cancers in the first few years, but since my sentinel lymph nodes were spared, Dr. G felt I had a good shot at avoiding that.

It always made me shudder to observe a "newbie" settling down in the chemo chair for first time, eyes darting around the room to observe the nurses and the equipment and the rest of us in our various stages of health. I knew what they were thinking. "What am I doing here?" It doesn't take long before you feel like a chemo room veteran.

You don't soon forget the face of the young man with advanced liver cancer who is just trying to buy a little more time, or the thirty-something woman with the mutated BRCA gene fighting triple-negative breast cancer that has metastasized – her two young daughters weighing heavily on her mind. And you never forget to appreciate life.

With the end of chemotherapy actually within my grasp, I could imagine feeling a bit better by July. I could imagine eating and tasting good food. The taste of food adds so much zest to life and I couldn't wait grasp that zest again!

Soon, I knew, I would likely be told that for all modern medicine could tell, I was cancer-free. Soon, it would be time to recover and celebrate.

Since the day I first found that lump, one of the reasons I remained strong was because of the doctors and nurses who became such an important part of my life. Fighting cancer takes a team, and I lucked into an amazing group of medical professionals who treated Jim and me as people who just happen to be fighting cancer.

While counting down the weeks until the end of chemotherapy, we continued working feverishly on completing *No More Secs!* The cover, the set up, the formatting, the planning...it's a time-consuming process. For me, doing that while in the throes of chemo fog was a huge challenge, especially given the fact that I did not want to admit to chemo fog.

Jim had so many hats to wear, so many balls to juggle, that working on getting the book published was nothing short of a labor of love. He spent time he didn't have in order to give me something I so desperately wanted. He understood my need to see it through and accomplish this goal. He wanted me to achieve my modest dream.

When it came down to the second to last chemo, number 15, Dr. G again broached the topic of radiation treatment. Up until that point, Jim and I both had the impression that he was leaning toward skipping radiation. We were wrong. In retrospect, it was a good thing. Sixteen chemotherapy sessions over a period of almost six months was a lot to handle. Had we known about the next leg of the journey, it would have been that much more difficult to bear.

The aggressive nature of my tumor, and its location just a hair away from the chest wall, was of great concern. As it was explained to us, chemotherapy sometimes doesn't work as well at the surgical site, so radiation is a good added precaution. Due to the lack of substance left in my chest, any future surgery there would prove difficult. We had to do all we could to ensure that would never be necessary.

Dr. G had already consulted with a radiation oncologist who suggested that a five-week course of radiation, given five days each week, would be the best course of action.

The good news was that they wanted to let me rest for three or four weeks after the final chemo before beginning radiation. That was also the bad news, as it would stretch treatment well into August. An appointment with the radiation oncologist was scheduled for the end of June.

While I had been gearing up to celebrate the end of more than half a year of chemo, my mood suddenly dampened. The thought of beginning a new long phase of treatment that would take up part of every weekday overwhelmed me. I was so sick and tired of being sick and tired. Would this never end?

I feared that once the effects of chemo wore off and I started to feel like myself, it would be very difficult to begin treatment again. In my heart of hearts, I knew I must continue. Dr. G. made a strong case. The battle to prevent recurrence was a crucial one. Fighting cancer a second time would be more difficult. If cancer did come back, we'd fight just as hard, but we didn't want to live with the regret of not having done all we could the first time around. It was that simple.

Whenever I began to feel down, I thought about my MS. How fortunate I was that it was still in remission!

"Look, she's got a cane!" He laughed as he said it, thinking it was some sort of prop. Then he noticed I was actually using the cane to walk ever so slowly across the parking lot. He turned away, unable to meet my gaze as his faux pas hung in the air like a bubble above a cartoon character's image. The thought of responding was all too exhausting. I needed to focus my energy on making it to the entrance with dignity. Like a housecat who suddenly finds herself out in the wide-open spaces, I longed for the security of walls and objects on which to brace myself.

It was a day to remember. Like Thanksgiving and Christmas and the fourth of July all rolled into one glorious celebration. It was Tuesday, June 7, 2011 and I was about to receive chemotherapy for the 16th and final time. Six long months of this cancer-fighting poison coursing through my veins was about to end. Sixteen times, we sat in that room. Sixteen times, I felt the medications surging through my body; 16 times, I felt the symptoms crash upon me in waves;

16 times, Jim and I slogged our way through the fog; 16 times, we did this thing in the hope that it would save my life. We were tired and more than ready to wrap it up in a big pink bow and put it behind us.

Of course, I'd have to get through two or three more weeks of feeling lousy, but from that point in the road, it would feel like a cakewalk.

My blood work was borderline, but with the doctor's approval, we proceeded as planned. It was a good session. As was my pattern, I fell into and out of sleep at first, then read and watched my feet swell to double their usual size. As I pushed my IV pole toward the restroom, I knew I would not miss the room, or its sights and smells. I would not miss the metal taste as the medication hit my system, and I would not miss having my chemo port poked. I would not miss the anxiety as my blood was checked to see if I was up to another round just yet. I would not miss the feeling of setting up the next appointment, or of walking out the door knowing that in a few days, the ill effects would wash over me and permeate every pore.

I would not miss seeing Jim stoically sitting in the chair next to me, contemplating who knows what while staring at his Kindle.

I would miss something, though I couldn't quite put my finger on it. Was it the other patients? Hard to say. There were so many and we came and went at different intervals, so there was no continuity in who we saw. The nurses? They were always so busy, yet so professional and caring.

The nurse explained that it's not unusual for chemo patients to experience a wide range of emotions, from elation to depression, in the weeks and months that follow the final treatment. After months of fighting cancer, suddenly you stop fighting, and that can make you feel rather helpless and anxious.

I felt strangely excited, anticipating life outside the confines of chemotherapy. On the other hand, any elation I might have felt was tempered by the fact that my fight was not yet over. I had a lengthy schedule of radiation therapy looming. It was not yet an ending; it was just a bend in the road.

"I'll see you in six months," said Dr. G with a smile. I liked the guy, I really did, but I sincerely hoped I would have no need to see him sooner.

After the IV was removed from my port and we were sent on our way, we felt the urge to mark the occasion in some way. Since Mexican food was one of the few types I could actually taste, we headed off to have a midday meal at our favorite Mexican restaurant. It was our way of marking the bend, and nothing else was required.

CHAPTER 14

No More Secs!

When it comes right down to it, you don't spend a lot of time with your doctors. When you're faced with long-term care, you come to depend on nurses. Their demeanor and expertise have a direct impact on your health and your state of mind. Nurses are on the front lines, right alongside you.

Our main experience with nurses is generally at the doctor's office. They greet us and lead us to the examining room. They ask questions and take our blood pressure and weight. They are a part of the routine easily overlooked in the shuffle, as we patients concern ourselves with making good use of our time with the doctor and the mundane matters of health insurance.

Then comes the health crisis – the big injury, the life-threatening illness, the trip to the hospital – and everything changes. Nurses suddenly become a very important part of our lives, and they have the power to change everything about how we cope with that crisis.

For me, triple-negative breast cancer is the crisis that pushed nurses into the spotlight of my health care. From the first visit to my breast surgeon's office, through surgery and other hospital procedures, and throughout chemotherapy, nurses were our main point of contact.

They were the ones who double and triple checked to make sure I received the correct medications in just the right doses. In between doctor visits, nurses answered my questions and gave advice on how to overcome side effects without prescription medications. They shared the little secrets about how to get more comfortable or how to work around a problem.

Above and beyond the call of duty, nurses asked what my weekend plans were, what book I was reading, and if I saw the latest movie. They chatted me up or touched my hand to distract from less pleasant happenings. They intuitively offered blankets and something to drink just when I needed them.

Nursing is a profession that comes with awesome responsibilities and a high level of stress. Despite that, most nurses manage to treat their patients with dignity, responding to their emotions as well as their physical symptoms.

Sometimes the simple act of looking a patient in the eye and offering a smile is all it takes to make that difference. So, I offer a heartfelt thank you to all the nurses who made a difference in my life during my treatment for cancer.

That thank you extends beyond my own treatment, because I've had the good fortune to observe nurses tending to others. Thank you to nurses who dispense hugs to patients who seem so alone; to nurses who put their own troubles aside in order to care for others; to nurses who stay a little longer and work a little harder because of staffing shortages; to nurses who remain calm despite the chaos that sometimes erupts around them; to nurses who keep doing what they do, day after day and year after year. It takes a certain kind of dedication and purpose to do what they do.

I want those nurses to know that what they do matters. Even though I can't remember all their names, I remember their faces. I remember their eyes. I remember their kindness. That kindness is as powerful as the medicine they practice.

My online articles about life with breast cancer generated some very different opinions. In spite of the negative backlash, some people went so far as to call me a hero, or brave.

Some called my scars a badge of honor.

I respectfully disagree. I'm not so brave. To me, bravery is putting your own best interests aside for someone else or for the greater good. I didn't volunteer for anything – I was drafted – and I did what I had to do to stay alive. There are so many who carry much greater burdens than my own. But I have learned that I'm a lot stronger of will and of spirit than I thought, and there is no shortage of supportive and caring people in this world.

Once chemotherapy was over, that handy little chemo port would have to be removed. Another surgery was scheduled to take place prior to the first radiation treatment. Considering everything I'd already been through, and all I was about to go through, this minor outpatient surgery wasn't of much consequence. Except that it was.

The chemo port was a security blanket of sorts, a way of protecting my stressed out veins. The act of removing it gave me a feeling of increased vulnerability, as though chemotherapy may be needed again at any moment and I would not be prepared. Chemotherapy was such a big part of my life that it felt inconceivable that I could be entirely free of it.

So many thoughts go through your mind when you experience these things. Like everyone else, Jim and I had responsibilities that would not go away just because I had cancer. As freelancers, every hour spent in treatment was an hour that we were not earning or pitching a new gig. Eventually, it begins to catch up with you.

Whether it's MS, cancer, or some other major health issue, there's a definite ripple effect in your life, extending from the physical to employment to health insurance to your social life, and it touches everyone around you. It's an invisible symptom of illness largely unnoticed by people who haven't lived it.

Two days after that last chemo, as side effects raged and June weather brought the sunshine, Jim completed the painstaking job of hand-coding the manuscript of *No More Secs!* for e-book format. He uploaded it to the publishing platform, filled in all the necessary information, and was ready to roll.

I stood behind him as he sat at his computer, holding the cursor over the publish button. "Ready?"

I was more than ready, but a little apprehensive as well. Publishing a memoir is like wearing your heart on your sleeve for all the world to see. It takes a willingness to share personal thoughts and experiences on a world stage. For an introvert like me, that's quite a leap.

"Ready."

No More Secs! made its official debut on June 9, 2011, and I was alive to see it happen. Ready or not, world, here it comes. What a way to pull yourself from the chemo doldrums!

I busied myself with fierce book promotion in addition to my other writing. It was the perfect segue into the eye of the storm between chemo and radiation. With each sale of a book, and with each email or comment from a stranger, I was reminded why I wrote the book in the first place. I was touching a nerve, reaching people in a way I never had before. From somewhere deep within me emerged a renewed sense of enthusiasm and purpose, and the resulting energy made the rest of June fly by.

Just as I was beginning to appreciate the freedom from ongoing chemotherapy, we had a meeting with my radiation oncologist. His office was located in the same building and even on the same floor as Dr. G. The same large entryway. The same smell of Subway to greet me. The same people roaming the corridors. The same mixture of hope and fear in the air. The same feeling of never-endingness.

As expected, Dr. S recommended a regimen of 25 treatments to take place five days a week for five weeks.

The radiation decision was not an easy one. Who the heck wants radiation? I certainly didn't. But this doctor impressed upon us that the tumor was dangerously close to my lung and that if any cancer cells remained behind, it would be a bad situation. He was also concerned about the positioning of the tumor. It was located so high on my breast that even though the lymph nodes under my arm were cancer-free, it was possible that cancer cells could have migrated to the lymph nodes behind my collar bone. Why hadn't I thought of that before?

It was the consensus of my medical team that radiation would be an important part of the overall plan to prevent recurrence or spread of triple-negative breast cancer. Surgery and chemotherapy were over, but the seriousness of my particular case was not something any of us could ignore.

Decisions regarding breast cancer treatment can be confusing and intimidating. It is wise to seek out the opinions of doctors. It is fair to request and welcome input of trusted family members and friends. But ultimately, these decisions belong to the patients, for we must be able to live with them.

How many decisions had I made since finding that breast lump? Too many to count. From deciding to see a doctor immediately, to following a fast track course to diagnosis, to consciously accepting the medical team that seemed to form itself around me, the decisions came quickly, but not without careful consideration.

Lumpectomy or mastectomy? Reconstructive surgery or prosthetic breast? Chemotherapy? Chemo port? Radiation? Drugs to combat individual symptoms or side effects? Complementary or alternative treatment? Diet, rest, exercise, general lifestyle, patient support groups, clinical trials...not to mention job, family, and social obligations. It's enough to make your head spin.

Dr. S wanted the chemo port removed before starting radiation, so on June 30th, I had the outpatient surgical procedure to remove it. Some of the same nurses who took care of me when it was inserted were there to do so again, and they remembered me.

Unfortunately, they couldn't use the chemo port to give

me an IV. The veins in my left arm were visibly damaged during the early days of chemotherapy and I suffered another blown vein. After a few tries, the nurses wanted to get an ultrasound to help them find a good vein. I was all for it because my arm was throbbing and the ultrasound machine worked for me in the past. Jim was all for it because the process was excruciating to watch.

The surgeon, whom I'd never met before, had other ideas. He overruled the nurses, insisting I had plenty of good veins to tap into. He directed them to try again. Another try, more pain, another failure.

By the time the doctor relented and called for an ultrasound, my arm was a bruised mess. Finally, they accessed a vein and we could move on.

That "twilight" sleep thing is quite a trip, but at least I could fade off. I hated that feeling of going under the anesthetic, knowing that Jim must play the waiting game once again. When I woke up, I was port free, with just a few stitches on my upper chest.

Removing the chemo port marked the end of an era, one I hoped never to revisit. I was beginning to enjoy the taste of food once again, just in time for those glorious summer veggies and fruits. I savored each morsel of food as though I'd never tasted anything like it before.

I found myself singing more often, in my usual off-key style, a sure sign that I was feeling better.

My world was in transition again.

CHAPTER 15

Lucy with a Mustache

When you're going to have radiation treatments, you have to get what they call "marked." That could very well be the most important part of the whole thing, and it's not a procedure that can be rushed.

The radiation team arranged me on a table. They moved my arm here, adjusted my chest there, ever so slightly this way or that. There was a lot of discussion, measuring, and generous amounts of black marker. I looked like a kindergarten art project gone wrong.

After everyone was in agreement that the marks were in the correct place, it was time to get permanently marked. In other words, it was time to get tattooed. Me! Tattooed! I got 10 tattoos, 10 little black dots strategically placed over the right side of my chest for all time.

The tattoos serve multiple functions. First, the dots help the team isolate the correct location for each session to make sure they're hitting the right spot and not endangering nearby tissues. Second, radiation generally isn't repeated in the same area, so should I ever have cancer again, the tattoos will tell doctors exactly where I've already had radiation. I was in for a strange five weeks. Radiation is nothing like chemotherapy, but it shares that *Twilight Zone* effect.

I didn't like the new tattoos on my previously unadorned body. They're so high that even with a conservative top, some show. They look like little black freckles. They tried to tell me that my new tattoos were a badge of honor that I survived cancer, but I wasn't buying it. Again with the badge of honor? Why do people feel the need to prop cancer patients up with this stuff? I didn't do anything to feel honored about. It's not like I threw myself in front of a bus to save a baby. Surviving cancer treatment? I just consider myself fortunate...grateful...eager to move on. I deserve no honor for simply surviving. If anything, the tattoos represent my gratefulness for those who treated me, and those who supported me emotionally, for Jim, and for David, Liz, and Tommy. Maybe they should have a badge of honor.

I no longer wish to escape the tattoos. They serve as a reminder of how close I came to losing my life. Just a few more weeks without noticing the lump, just a month's hesitation, any delay in getting an appointment could have changed everything.

My tattoos, like my scars, tell the story of me.

I was scheduled for my first radiation treatment the following Monday. In the meantime, I needed to go back to the hospital to have the stitches removed from my chest. I wasn't allowed to get the stitches wet, so having them removed meant nice, long morning showers again, no small matter.

After the stitches were out, I headed toward my car. While in the parking lot, I heard someone calling my name. A nurse was jogging toward me, hair flying behind her and a big smile on her face. "I meant to tell you before you left. I'm reading your book. I'm on chapter four and I love it! I just wanted you to know."

A fan! My first fan! Tattoos in place, stitches out, and I had a fan! What a glorious day! How kind of her to make the effort. It doesn't always seem like it, but the world does have a good share of kind people.

How ironic that as I navigated through cancer treatment, my book about life with MS was beginning to find readers. The MS that was taking a back seat to cancer. The MS that was still in remission. How long could it last, I wondered.

Following cancer treatment, would it return with a vengeance, or would it allow me more time to build up my strength?

In the days that followed, I finally began to get my taste buds back. Full flavor still eluded me, but at least things tasted somewhat like I remembered. Salad, salmon, cantaloupe, and a host of foods reappeared on my favorites list. Things were looking up.

Not all the symptoms of chemo were willing to exit the scene. My teary-eye problem showed no signs of letting up, my feet still doubled in size by the end of each day, and I still saw nothing but scalp on the top of my head.

Eyebrows and eyelashes stubbornly refused to come to life, yet I needed to shave my legs. Go figure. The universe definitely has a sense of humor.

We generally think of eyelashes as mere decoration, but as I tried to enjoy a little excursion into the backyard each afternoon, I discovered just how useful eyelashes are. The backyard gnats insisted on flitting about my face and, with nothing to get in the way, collided with my eyeballs at every opportunity. I couldn't blink fast enough to rid myself of the little pests. Drat. Instead of relaxing and catching a few rays, I flailed about wildly, making a complete spectacle of myself.

That's the kind of thing that brought out a touch of anger. Like the head cold before surgery, the gnats ruining my afternoons outside totally pissed me off.

The worst thing of all, though, was that I'd become a complete stranger to people who should have known me. I used to dismiss those episodes of *I Love Lucy* where Ricky didn't recognize his own wife because she put on a cowboy hat or glued a mustache under her nose. And how come Lois Lane couldn't recognize Superman just because he wore glasses when in his Clark Kent persona? Come on, now, that couldn't happen.

Yet, it happened to me. I wore a cap instead of hair and was light on the eyebrows and eyelashes, but people who should have known me didn't. I could understand it if my identity didn't register as we passed on the street. It was worse than that, though.

I found it unsettling that complete strangers could take one look at me and feel compelled to offer life advice, while people I'd met before could not or would not look at me.

There were times I stood by Jim's side as he engaged in conversation with folks who barely acknowledged my existence.

Jim didn't bother to introduce us, because we'd been introduced before. We'd had conversations and they'd heard my voice. They knew me to be Jim's wife. If they didn't recognize me, why didn't they introduce themselves to me, or make eye contact? Why didn't they ask Jim who I was? As we parted, why did they always say it was nice to "meet" me? It doesn't get more *Twilight Zone* than that.

Did nothing about me give me away? My mannerisms, my voice, my facial expressions, the fact that I was standing next to Jim? This was the cruelest side effect of them all, for it caused me to question the very core of my being.

I was Lucy with a mustache. I could rob banks in broad daylight and get away with it.

I felt about as unremarkable and uninteresting as one can be, to be so unrecognizable as all that. As much he tried, Jim could not console me by pointing out the obvious – that my appearance was, in fact, different. To my mind, it was an indication that I – the inner essence of me – had failed to make an impression. The soul-searching would continue for a long time to come.

Five weeks of radiation loomed and if I was to move forward, I needed to have a heart-to-heart talk with myself. It is my nature to turn to writing when it's time to dig deep, so write I did.

"Note to Self:

"I survived finding a breast lump, informing Jim, having a mammogram, an ultrasound, a double biopsy, and the shocking diagnosis of a fast growing, very aggressive triple-negative breast cancer. I survived informing my family by long distance.

"I survived a mastectomy, the drain, the stitches, and the physical and emotional healing of losing a breast.

"I survived four rounds of Adriamycin (the Red Devil) and Cytoxan and their sometimes hellish side effects, including going completely bald, anemia, weight loss, blown veins, and fatigue. I survived having a chemo port surgically inserted into my chest.

"I survived 12 rounds of Taxotere and a host of unpleasant side effects, including extreme fatigue, continuing anemia, a constant flow of tears from my eyes, blood leaking from my nose...and other places. I survived the delays due to poor blood work and a need to rest my tired body before slamming it again.
I survived the waiting, the doctors' appointments, the decisions, and the stranger in the mirror.

"I survived the haunting stories of my fellow cancer patients, feeling their anguish as keenly as my own.

"I survived more than half a year of chemotherapy with my positive attitude intact. I continued to work, even taking on additional writing jobs. I took a road trip to celebrate Mom's 80th birthday, one to share Easter with Jim's family, and another to witness Liz's college graduation. Although I did less, I continued to cook dinner almost every night, and managed at least something in the way of household chores every week.

"I survived watching Jim bravely carry unspoken burdens on his strong shoulders.

"I will survive the 25 doses of radiation and whatever side effects they bring because it is what I must do. This is still the all-important war to prevent recurrence. When it is over, I will know that I did all I could. If it recurs anyway, I will be stronger for that knowledge.

"I survived and will continue to survive because I'm not done living.

"I survived and will continue to survive because David, Liz, and Tommy give me strength and love and they're not ready to lose their mother. My family has rallied around and they shouldn't have to say goodbye yet.

"I survived and will continue to survive because I am married to Jim. Our love is one for the ages, and we're not ready to be separated. I survive because Jim walks every step with me, loving me and accepting each change as it comes. We survive because Team Pietrangelo is outrageously stubborn and strong where that love is concerned, and never passes up an opportunity to prove it. We survive because it is what we do and who we are.

"We survive because we did not stop living after diagnosis, or surgery, or chemotherapy, or the thought of radiation, or weariness, and we will never stop living as long as we're together. Our pleasures are simple and our needs are few, but they are ours to enjoy. We will survive and thrive, together, as long as we *live*."

I inserted a chart of the upcoming radiation schedule so I could put an "X" next to each day when I returned home. I plastered that note to self front and center on the refrigerator door. I would look at it each morning, as a reminder of what we'd already accomplished and how much we had to look forward to.

I had my very own little power meeting and prepared to face the next five weeks of radiation therapy with a healthy dose of respect for the process, eager to hear another doctor say, "see you in six months."

CHAPTER 16

The Radiation Zone

Monday, July 11 arrived and it was time to enter the radiation zone. I imagined there should be alarms, blinking lights, and HAZMAT suits. Radiation seemed like something to avoid, rather than something you willingly do to yourself. It's all a matter of perspective.

After six months of accompanying me to treatment, it wasn't easy for Jim to let go. After much discussion, he agreed that it wasn't necessary to accompany me to radiation treatment. It wasn't worth wasting his time each day when he would only be sitting in the waiting room, anyway.

It was explained that the actual radiation treatment would take only about 10 minutes and that I should be in and out within 45 minutes. Side effects generally begin slowly and build over time. They might include dryness, itching, peeling, or reddening of the skin. The worst side effect, by most accounts, would be fatigue as the weeks wore on. That turned out to be the understatement of the century.

As with the chemotherapy oncology office, the waiting room for radiation oncology had a fair number of people, most of them waiting for a patient to return from the inner office. This cancer thing is entirely too prevalent.

After signing in, I was directed to a dressing room where I was to remove my shirt and bra and put on a hospital gown. Then I joined a line of similarly gowned people waiting their turn in chairs placed along the walls. There was even less interaction between patients here than there was in chemotherapy. That's because none of us stayed in one place very long. We went from the outer waiting room to a private dressing room to a chair in the hallway to the treatment room and back. There were several treatment rooms and teams of technicians keeping things running about as on time as any medical facility I've ever encountered.

I was asked to lie flat on the table while equipment was adjusted and the room readied. Even with tattoos, correct positioning is an art form. The head and arms must be just so. A wedge pillow behind the knees helps keep you comfortable and in position. The table moves and the equipment moves, but for the patient, remaining still is the number one job. Actually, it's the only job.

One wall of the room was lined with lush plants and a small water fountain intended to give patients something to look at during treatment, I suppose. Unfortunately, I was positioned with my face turned to the left, toward a shelving unit that contained masks, torsos, and other body part molds marked with patients' names.

I learned that these are used to keep patients from moving, especially those who are receiving radiation to the head or face. I wondered who wore them and how they felt when they put them on. I'm not claustrophobic, but I was grateful I didn't need anything like that. The facemasks stared back at me like ghosts seeking confirmation of their existence. I half expected them to make a move toward me or ask me to help them escape their prison.

The technicians were wonderful and made an effort to keep up pleasantries as they moved various parts of my body. "Just let yourself go and let us do the moving." That's a little bit harder to do than you might think. Letting go isn't easy.

The actual radiation treatments are painless and if it's not hard for you to keep still, it's not a bad experience. It soon became a matter of routine. Get up. Eat breakfast. Shower. Dress. Drive to radiation therapy. Back to work. My life was structured around daily treatment, but it was a smooth operation. It is a true testament to the human spirit that we can constantly adapt when we are properly motivated. And motivated I was. This was it. The last leg of the journey to beat cancer back into submission. The final battle in the war over the body in which I must live. At least that was my hope. I couldn't have gone through it if I didn't believe it was the right thing to do.

My eyelashes wanted to grow back, they really did, but they apparently didn't know which way was up. A few of the nasty little hairs were growing straight down and repeatedly stabbing me in the eyes, which only exacerbated my teary-eye syndrome. I really and truly wanted eyelashes, but getting stabbed in the eye was getting on my nerves.

One day, in a fit of exasperation, I actually plucked a couple of eyelashes right out of my upper lids. Relief at last. I wonder if that had something to do with the fact that nothing ever grew back in those spaces. You probably shouldn't follow my lead in the whole eyelash-plucking thing. A little patience goes a long way.

Relapsing/remitting MS is a mysterious thing. Symptoms come and go. You can go from being unable to walk for a month to participating in a five-mile Walk MS event the next.

Serious symptoms of MS began to plague me in the summer of 2003 and although I had brief remissions, it changed everything about my life. Along with having to find a new way to earn a living, MS caused my living expenses to rise dramatically, especially where health insurance was concerned. Once you fall out of group coverage, and once you use up your allotted time paying through COBRA, you find yourself in the land of the death spiral health insurance policy. You take the highest deductible allowed, you do your best to keep up with ever-rising premiums, and you do everything in your power to NOT seek medical attention. It's a ridiculous system. As premiums rise, the healthier participants opt out, leaving only the sickest, which leads to higher premiums, which leads to...well, you get the picture.

Some cancer patients who were treated alongside me came from many miles away. Some drove several hours each way every day for their treatment. How in the world could those people hang on to their jobs? What would happen to them when they lost their livelihood and their health insurance right along with it?

I wish more people understood or cared about the insanity of it all and the burdens we place on the people who become ill. Let's face it. Nobody is immune to the need for health care.

Cancer was a more immediate threat to my life, but MS changed everything about how I function in this world. Each disease comes with its own set of challenges.

One of the most puzzling and amazing things about all this is that my MS was still in remission. Why? I wish I knew. Did the cancer alter my immune system and shake things up? Did the chemotherapy knock the wind out of its sails? The doctors I've spoken with are loath to offer a theory, and I can hardly blame them. If you've got to have a mystery in your life, a dormant disease is good one to have.

Within a year, minor symptoms of MS would reappear, mostly in the form of muscle spasms. They started in my fingers and toes, and then graduated to my feet and lower legs. Sometimes the muscles in my abdomen spasm, but it never lasts long or causes great inconvenience. The major symptoms that formerly pummeled away at me – crushing fatigue, inability to walk, inability to use my arms – remain at bay. Mobility aids I once depended on are, for now, unnecessary.

I don't kid myself that my MS is cured. I fully understand that many people with relapsing/remitting MS go years, even decades, between relapses. I'm grateful that I am now among them. Should it return, I will be disappointed, but not surprised. I will simply have to learn to live with it and around it again.

In the meantime, I'll enjoy my modestly robust health and try to keep my body strong.

CHAPTER 17

The Plot Thickens

I never could tell the difference between honeybees, hornets, wasps, yellow jackets, bumblebees, or other such buzzing creatures, so I just refer to them all as bees.

It is often said that if you don't bother the bees, they won't bother you, but that hasn't been my experience. I've been stung three times just standing around minding my own business. I never even saw them coming. That's why I turned into one of those crazy people who go a little wild in the presence of the little buzzers.

David was playing outside and dropped half a banana on the hot concrete of the patio. I didn't notice it until it began attracting bees. Lots of them. Oh, great. Now our little patio/play area is filling up with bees! I've got to do something about this before one of the kids gets stung. It was one of those parental moments when you have to pretend to be fearless when all you want to do is run away.

I carefully navigated my way around the bee/banana obstacle course and grabbed the end of the garden hose. I backed into the house through the patio door, handing the hose to David and closing the door enough so only the hose could fit through.

"David, this is what I want you to do. We're going to fight the bees on Banana Hill." He smirked, but was happy to play along with the game.

"You're going to spray the hose at the banana and keep the spray coming. When the bees fly away, I'll grab the banana." I was General Mom, leading the army into battle.

"Okay, Soldier. Ready...set...go!"

David let the stream fly and the bees scattered. As soon as the coast was clear, I swooped in and grabbed the remnants of the banana. I took the hose from David, cleaned up the concrete, and went inside. I was in fast motion, lest the bees return for revenge.

"Thank you, Soldier. Job well done." We exchanged snappy salutes.

Henceforth, our adventure would be known as The Bee Battle on Banana Hill.

Bees are a healthy and productive part of our ecosystem, but I prefer to keep my distance. In a perfect world, they would do the same. Unfortunately for me, they decided to cross my personal boundaries that summer. That's when I learned that bees no longer held such power over me. I really did learn not to sweat the small stuff.

One morning, as I was settling into my car to go to radiation therapy, I noticed some bees hovering around my right side door, but didn't give it much thought. As I buckled up after treatment, I noticed a few more bees that appeared fascinated with the mirror on my passenger side door. Still, I wasn't in the mood to give it a whole lot of thought. I had a lot on my mind and I was tired. I needed to get going.

I played this game of ignorant bliss for a week or so, watching as a handful of bees followed me from home to radiation and back each day like my own personal entourage. How odd it was, I thought, that wherever I go, so go the bees. You'd think they would tire of the ride and give up on all the commotion of a home on wheels.

From my vantage point today, it seems so silly that I would do that for so long, but the present, more clearheaded me knows better than to judge past me who was going through cancer treatment.

Finally, enough of them were hanging around that I became concerned about my safety. What if they came inside the car while I was driving? The distraction could cause a major problem. I escaped death by cold, so let's not have death by bee, now.

My suspicions at last aroused me out of complacency. After pulling my car into its parking spot in front of our home, I watched for a few moments. Bees were traveling back and forth between the bushes and my side mirror. They obviously had no intention of altering their routine.

It's not hard to figure out why they chose my car. It was always parked right in front of their home base. During the worst of my MS relapses, that car sat in place for weeks on end as Jim drove me to and from work. For the most part, we used Jim's car for errands and road trips. If cars had feelings, mine would have felt lonely and neglected. And probably invaded, as well.

As far as I was concerned, the whole bee thing was a job for Jim, one he willingly took on.

As the end of July came into view, the family decided to throw a birthday party for Jim's mother. To attend, we'd have to leave for New Jersey after my treatment on a Friday and return on Sunday so I could make my Monday morning appointment. It was going to be a quick in, a nice little party, and a quick out. My exhaustion was growing and I was worn out just thinking about it.

If there's one thing Jim and I can attest to, it's that things don't always go according to plan. You can make all the plans you want, but be prepared for alterations.

A few days before the party, Mom was injured in a car accident, necessitating a trip to the emergency room followed by a few days in the hospital. Instead of a road trip and a party, Jim suddenly had more worry on his plate. He wanted to go to his mother's side, but he didn't want to leave me all alone while I was going through radiation treatment.

While other family members tended to Mom, Jim stayed with me. Then the plot thickened. That Sunday, he awoke with a pain in his lower abdomen, a pain he managed to live with for a few hours before mentioning it. Jim has an extremely high tolerance for pain. He's never had a major surgery or spent a single day in a hospital.

It was Sunday, so he wanted to wait until Monday to call the doctor. When he reached his pain threshold and could hold out no longer, he was ready to admit that something was terribly wrong. When he finally agreed to go to the emergency room, I was greatly relieved, but more than a little worried.

The place was packed with people of all ages, though no one seemed particularly ill or injured. We jumped through the required hoops, handing over the insurance card and filling out the voluminous forms. We sat and waited several hours for our turn to be seen.

On the outside I was calm, but on the inside I was worried out of my mind. For Jim to drag himself there meant that something was terribly wrong. What if he was ill? What if he needed surgery or something? How could I possibly give him the care and support he deserved? I was barely keeping myself together.

After we were assigned to a bed, a nurse gave Jim an IV for fluids. The ER doc decided right off the bat that it couldn't be kidney stones because Jim would be in much worse pain. "What have you taken for pain?" the doctor wanted to know.

"Nothing."

"Do you want something for pain?"

"No."

"Are you sure? We can have you feeling better pretty fast."

"I'd rather wait until we know what's wrong."

"We're going to get you to a CT scan and find out what's going on."

After the doctor left, the nurse came back with a small vial of liquid and headed over to the IV pole.

"What's that?" asked Jim.

"Morphine."

"Morphine! I don't want any morphine!"

"But it'll relieve the pain."

"I haven't even had so much as an aspirin and you want to give me morphine? Get that away from me."

Maybe it was just my imagination, but I think the nurse looked a little dejected.

As they wheeled him away for the scan, I momentarily felt how I imagine Jim must have felt each time I was wheeled away for one procedure or another. It's no fun to be in pain or to be fighting cancer, but it's no picnic on the flipside, either. It's a terrible thing, to be left alone to ponder the implications of what may come. You hang on to a positive train of thought, but you know life doesn't always go your way and the possibilities bounce around your brain at warp speed.

The CT scan revealed a single, small kidney stone. After four hours in the ER, we walked out with a strainer and a prescription for pain medication.

Within an hour of arriving back home, Jim passed the stone without so much as a whimper. He never did fill the prescription.

I couldn't have been more relieved that the crisis had passed. Dealing with my treatment and Mom's injuries was more than enough for one man to handle.

The bill came to just shy of $4,000 and, because of our high deductible, it was entirely out-of-pocket. They don't offer morphine for that kind of pain.

A few days later, Jim's mother was recovering at home and it was his turn to help out. Of course, he wanted to, but he struggled with his choice. To drive to New Jersey and stay with his mother for a few days meant he'd be leaving me all alone.

Aside from fatigue, I was doing well enough and knew I could manage on my own. I understood why he needed to go and knew that he should go. I assured him that it was the right thing to do, even though I didn't want to be on my own. I wasn't as confident on the inside as I tried to appear on the outside.

What a terrible position to be in. Two people who need you are separated by a five-hour drive and still you must keep up with your own work so you can pay all the damned bills that never stop coming. And still, few people ever bothered to ask Jim how he was coping.

Smokey and I were left to our own devices for a few days. Jim alerted our next door neighbors and it was comforting to know they could come to my aid in a pinch. I made it to and from treatment, kept the house running, and worked feverishly on my writing. Just as he had kept phone tabs on Mom while he was with me, he kept phone tabs on me while he was away.

It felt strange, being alone while undergoing radiation treatment for cancer, with no next of kin around in case of emergency. I had a sense of isolation and could only hope that nothing else would happen to upset our delicate ecosystem.

The bees were back, buzzing around my car again, but I learned to tolerate their presence until Jim's return. Funny. Bees used to scare me silly, but I no longer gave in to that fear. Hey, when you're dealing with cancer, bees don't seem especially menacing. They're only insects, after all.

Maybe it's precisely because we didn't have family around that we remained so independent. It never occurred to us that we couldn't or shouldn't maintain a normal schedule. The support we had was emotional support, and it came from all across the country. More acquaintances and strangers than I can count sent good vibes our way. There's a lot to be said about that.

I hope I send out good vibes in return. I hope I never get

so comfortable as to pass up an opportunity to uplift someone in need.

CHAPTER 18

Moving the Goalposts

Each day, I placed an "X" on the calendar after treatment. I anxiously awaited the end of the daily ordeal and what I hoped would be a return to a somewhat normal life. But my radiation oncologist was not finished with me.

"I've been studying your file and I'd like to add one more week of treatment." Hell, no! He did not just say that! If heads really could explode, mine was on the verge of doing so.

His reasoning was compelling. It was the location of the tumor that had him concerned. He wanted to perform five more treatments that would be highly targeted to the small area where the large tumor was removed. Any remaining cancer cells could very well be in or dangerously close to the lymph nodes near my collarbone. One more week and he would feel that he did all he could. I could only hope there was nothing else to follow and the goalposts wouldn't move again.

Despite the fact that radiation would now be concentrated on that one small area, nothing else about the experience changed. I expanded the chart on my refrigerator and set my mind to finishing this thing.

By the time I reached that final week, my skin was extremely tender and pink. Exhaustion was setting in and it was becoming increasingly difficult to keep up with my workload.

Meanwhile, something was trying to sprout out of the top

of my head, but it didn't look like hair. It couldn't figure out what color it wanted to be. I grew brown hair, but there was also black, gray, white, and red. Little bits of hair growth managed to poke their way through the top of my head only to fall out again, leaving me with a patchwork quilt look. Since I no longer worked at the funeral home, I had little use for that stifling wig and it became the summer of the hat.

We needed something to look forward to in our After Cancer Life and didn't we deserve a break? We started scoping out excursions to warm, tropical islands and solicited pamphlets about European river cruises. We talked about our dream trip – Italy, a nod to Jim's heritage, and France, a nod to mine. We wanted to celebrate life and the fact that I still had one. But the toll of the previous year was heavy, and there was something else we wanted to do, perhaps a bit less glamorous, but a lot more important.

We outlined plans for yet another road trip. We would load up the Subaru and head toward Southern Illinois to visit with Liz, hoping David and Tommy could meet us down there. After a few days we would aim for New Orleans to visit with Jim's daughter. It would be a relaxing, no pressure road trip and a way to see some of our kids, not to mention a visit to one of our favorite cities in the world. It was what we both wanted and needed. The anticipation would give me the strength I needed to get through the final days of treatment.

The great part about the freelance life is that when we do travel, we can check in and respond to our clients. Sometimes, we can even fit in some small jobs when we're on the road.

It was one of our many fantasies – purchasing a mobile home equipped with the technology we needed to do our jobs while spending our days on the road. Not a bad dream, if taking care of a mobile home doesn't scare you off. I'm not sure we'd do well with that. I'm pretty sure it would be like something out of the movie, *RV*, or maybe *The Long, Long Trailer*. I just don't see it happening.

Catch That Look

On a sunny Friday morning in August, I showed up for my final radiation treatment. I hung my shirt and bra on the hook, complete with prosthetic breast, and donned the familiar robe. I sat and stared at my Kindle until my name was called. There were no surprises – no last minute reasons why I would need more treatment, no unanticipated twists or turns.

As the table was lowered to the point where I could sit up, the technician handed me a piece of paper. It was a diploma. I'd officially graduated from radiation.

We moms, and a couple of dads, waited outside the classroom. Our preschoolers were about to graduate, complete with colorful diplomas. The door opened and the teacher stepped out. From within the room came the strains of "Pomp and Circumstance," as each little one was called by name. A great whirring and clicking of video and still amateur photography filled the air. There were audible gasps and squeals of delight, as each mom caught sight of her child. A few children looked proud, but most appeared bewildered by the attention.

I dressed, placed the gown in the hamper, and pulled the flowered dressing room curtain aside. Diploma in one hand, purse in the other, I strolled through the half-filled waiting room and into the hallway. The aroma from Subway engulfed me, as it always did, but I realized with surprise that it no longer made me feel ill.

A strange feeling washed over me. I was, as far as I knew, finished with treatment. I was, as far as anyone knew, cancer-free, though no one officially declared it to be so.

I walked through the cavernous lobby toward the automatic doors, feeling for all the world like I was leaving one dimension and entering another. As I straddled these two worlds, I wasn't at all certain to which I belonged, or if I would find life on the other side recognizable.

Sunglasses were a must, but my eyes still watered as though I were crying. The sun felt good on my arms and a gentle wind made my army green skirt flutter around my knees. It was early in the day, so my feet had yet to swell within my comfy white sandals. I felt feminine. I felt strong and tentative at the same time, and slightly discombobulated.

I thought back to my first visit with Dr. M, when she called me a survivor. At the time, I didn't feel as though I'd survived anything out of the ordinary. Suddenly, I *felt* like a survivor...a warrior...a victor. I couldn't have done it without a lot of help, but I was still among the living and I had survived something BIG. At least a tiny fraction of that was due to my own effort, wasn't it?

The meaning of the word "survivor" suddenly became clear. It's about more than being alive. It's about being alive after walking through the fires of hell. Well, not hell exactly, but fire nonetheless. It's about walking that walk with purpose. It's about being alive in the moment, even when faced with an uncertain future. Suddenly, I understood what it means to be a true survivor.

Shouldn't such an occasion be met with crowds of well-wishers, streamers, and balloons? Where were the brass band, the fireworks, and the parade? Where were the reporters and photographers and heads of state? Shouldn't I be giving the royal wave as I stroll confidently through the excited throngs on the way to my waiting limo?

The only visible evidence of this monumental occasion was the paper diploma I'd already folded and stuffed inside my purse. I got in my car, opened the windows, and sat silently for a moment. I was a newly-released prisoner who passed through the giant metal gates with a new lease on life, not sure where to begin.

I opened up the sunroof, letting the sunshine and the warm summer air have their way with my head. This was going to be a great ride. With a nod to my entourage of bees, I cranked up the music and headed for home.

Jim greeted me with our customary hug and kiss, grateful

that we'd achieved another milestone. We were perfectly content with our quiet victory.

It was Friday, August 19, 2011. I reached for my calendar and made a final "X," beside which I wrote the word, "yay!"

The plan was that I would continue to see each doctor – the surgeon, the chemotherapy oncologist, and the radiation oncologist – each at six-month intervals, at least for the first two years. That way, multiple doctors would be checking up on me. That seemed sensible enough. There were no further imaging tests scheduled and I would have blood work every six months.

As fate would have it, it was time to visit with my surgeon, Dr. M, and she brought up a subject I'd dismissed before. Colonoscopy. It's not that I have anything against a colonoscopy, but come on! Enough is enough. I could spend my whole life doing one type of medical procedure or other. No! No! No! Couldn't I please go through one month without being poked and prodded like a lab specimen?

"But you're over 50," she said, "and you've already had cancer." She let me brush it aside once before, but she didn't want to drop it this time. She had a lot of persuasive arguments and I could fight her no longer. Fine. I'd have a colonoscopy. I made a vow to myself at that moment that this would end it. That's it. As long as my life was not at stake, I didn't want to go on an endless cycle of testing. I needed my freedom.

She recommended a doctor and we scheduled the colonoscopy for the second week of September. I wanted to get it out of the way so we could get on with our celebratory vacation.

The day before a colonoscopy is...well, let's just say it's awkward and unpleasant. You definitely don't want to leave the house. The colonoscopy itself is an outpatient procedure. Once again, Jim had to accompany me, watching and waiting while other people did things to me. It's not easy being him.

I hated the experience from the moment we stepped inside the cramped waiting room. The doctor was running hours behind. She wasn't even in the building and I was already tired, hungry, thirsty, and agitated by the idea of wasting the entire day when I should be getting on with my post-cancer life. I get very grouchy when I miss lunch.

As I changed into the gown, I was flooded with memories of surgery and radiation, just as I was beginning to put them behind me.

I hated having to take off my hat to reveal the ugly patches of hair that resembled scouring pads you might find under your kitchen sink. I hated leaving my bra and my fake breast behind, leaving me unbalanced again. I was a patient again, all too soon, and I wasn't taking it well.

I was told they'd be using the "twilight" sleep, which is not the same as general anesthesia. I'd had that several times before and never had a problem with it. "You're not going to need much of that," I told the doctor. "It hardly takes anything for me to go to sleep."

They gave me a dose and asked me if I was feeling sleepy. "Not yet," I said.

"Give her a little more," was the last thing I heard. Everything from that point until a day and a half later is a mystery to me. As it turned out, they gave me something that causes a bit of amnesia. Why should I need amnesia? Did you take me up into your flying saucer, pull out a probe, and do unspeakable things to me? Oh, right...

The next thing I recall is waking up on my living room sofa, sitting straight up, with a mouthful of macaroni. How long was I asleep, and how long was this food in my mouth? I didn't remember making any macaroni, much less eating it.

I made my way into the kitchen and noticed some paperwork on the counter. It was my hospital release and discharge instructions, complete with my own signature. I didn't recall ever seeing it before.

Jim went over the details with me. "Don't you remember leaving the hospital?"

"No. Did they wheel me out?"

"No. You walked out, but I knew you were out of it. Do you remember feeling like you were going to throw up?"

I had a faint, blurry flash of memory, a vision of myself picking up a small trash can in the hospital and telling him I needed to vomit into it. It was all I could piece together.

"I don't remember yesterday...what time is it? I don't even remember today. Was the colonoscopy okay? Did they find anything?"

Realizing the extent of my memory loss, Jim filled me in on the details. I had a perfectly normal colonoscopy result. Not the tiniest hint of cancer or another other problem. Well, that was good news, anyway.

CHAPTER 19

Michael Corleone and Me

As September progressed, so did I. My appetite and energy levels were showing signs of great improvement and I was busy with work. Jim was also finalizing the publication of *No More Secs!* in paperback format. It was a genuine pleasure to be free from the constraints of daily treatment and the side effects that go with it. I was free!

We firmed up the details of our road trip, which we planned for September 26 through October 5, during which time we would both celebrate our birthdays.

With our neighbor scheduled to keep any eye on Smokey, we loaded up the Subaru and headed out into the world once again, far from my doctors and all those things that reminded us cancer. My MS was still in remission and there was nothing, aside from lingering fatigue, to keep us from enjoying every moment. This was time we would not squander, for even on our best days, we were keenly aware of how quickly things can change.

Bright and early on a truly fabulous Monday morning, we started out on the first leg of our journey, which would take us from the Shenandoah Valley to Lexington, Kentucky. We left Virginia full of chatter, then settled into alternately listening to and singing along with the radio. The steady motion of the car lulled me into a semi-sleep more than once, but we enjoyed the very idea of being away, as if we were driving away from cancer and all its side effects. This trip wasn't a temporary relief from treatment; this one was a celebration that treatment was over.

We stopped for lunch, then for dinner, before reaching Lexington. I, for one, was pooped, and wanted to get as much rest as I could before we arrived in Illinois.

The next morning, we started out for Carbondale, Illinois. David would be unable to join us on this trip, but Tommy would meet us there. Only a few months had passed since Liz's graduation, but they would see a stronger-looking version of me.

I was still thin, but eating with renewed enthusiasm. There was nothing to stop me from enjoying three fun-filled, no stress days. The final day of our Illinois visit was Jim's birthday, so Liz and her boyfriend prepared a cozy dinner before we said our teary goodbyes. They were sad tears, because I would miss them so. They were contented tears, because they were able to see that I'd come out on the other side of this thing. They were happy tears, because sometimes life truly does go your way, and grants a precious favor. And, of course, there were those constant tears that seem to be a permanent feature of my life since chemo.

As part of our celebratory victory lap, we drove straight from Carbondale to Memphis, where we'd spend an afternoon and evening by ourselves. Jim wanted to do this up right, so he booked a lovely hotel room in the heart of Memphis. He arranged for us to be greeted with chocolates and champagne before embarking on a horse-drawn carriage tour of the city. What fun!

Our tour guide, Mary, was a character, one I swore I would use in a novel some day. Only I'd call her Hermione. It suits her better. She wore a flowing skirt, sneakers, and a wide-brimmed straw hat with a pink flower flopping lazily off to one side. Her carriage was covered in glitter, which clung to our shoes and clothing.

With a flair for the dramatic, she showed us around town, pointing out things of interest and referring to the "Yankees" of the Civil War period in her thick British accent. As she was facing forward in an open carriage and not using a microphone, we only caught bits and pieces of her spiel. Nevertheless, her enthusiasm was remarkable and I couldn't help but wonder about her backstory.

Mary was everything a horse-drawn carriage tour guide should be, and that's why I remember her so vividly.

As evening set in, Mary let us off in front of our hotel. After a quick change, we set out on foot to explore downtown Memphis before dinner. The rich sounds of music poured from every open doorway and just strolling the area was an experience.

We had a reservation at BB King's famous restaurant and planned a long, relaxed dinner. A spicy aroma filled the air. I savored the seasonings and relished the textures. I sipped my wine ever so slowly, as we soaked in the music and the energy of the room. Everyone was there for a good time.

We were about as far from the chemotherapy room as we could be, but even as I enjoyed the experience, I was drawn back to that room. It was evening, so all would be quiet. But in the morning, it would be humming along again at full speed, of that I was sure. The TVs would blare, patients would be hooked up to IVs and monitors, and nurses would be drawing blood, answering questions, and dispensing medication.

I was out, but it wasn't going to end. More people would be diagnosed and more would begin treatment each day. I owed it to them to appreciate my own good fortune and to be in the moment.

We made it. We really made it to the other side. Both aware of the high rate of recurrence for triple-negative breast cancer, we chose to focus on the present and not borrow trouble from what may come. This was surviving at its finest. This was thriving. This was the living, laughing, and loving part for sure. If I got nothing more than the pleasure of that road trip, it would be enough to make the previous year worth every poke, prod, pain, and platitude.

On Saturday morning, we set out for New Orleans to visit with Jim's daughter and celebrate my 52nd birthday. New Orleans is an amazing city with an unmatched flair for a good time. With my MS still in remission and my body recovering from all the trauma of the previous months, I had no trouble walking the city or taking full advantage of the tantalizing cuisine of New Orleans.

Jim's daughter treated us to dinner at a charming new restaurant on my birthday and we enjoyed every moment of our all-too-brief visit. By Tuesday, we were headed back to Virginia with a stopover in Chattanooga.

It was during this final leg of the journey that I began to feel a pain in the ass. Literally. My coccyx, more commonly known as the tailbone, was hurting and it was getting more and more difficult to sit without pain. I didn't give it much thought at first, although I shifted endlessly in my attempt to find a spot that didn't hurt. Now what?

Before Cancer, that was exactly the type of thing I would want to ignore, the type of thing sure to prompt expensive tests and lead nowhere. But I was living in After Cancer World, a place where any ache or pain could mean that cancer was making a comeback. Still, after a 10-day road trip, a sore behind wasn't entirely uncalled for.

Was the brief vacation from cancer and doctors over already? Would I be back in the cancer wars before my hair even grew back?

A week later, when the pain showed no sign of letting up, I made the call I didn't want to make. I explained my symptoms to a nurse at my oncologist's office and she promised to speak to the doctor.

The next day, I received a call from the hospital. Per my doctor's instructions, they wanted to set an appointment for an X-ray and a full-body bone scan. That could only mean one thing – my doctor was suspicious. No longer able to dismiss any medical test as inconsequential, my celebratory mood was dampened. More tests, another wait for answers, and another opportunity to receive bad news.

I was instructed to arrive at the hospital early in the morning to have some radioactive material injected into by body. Again with this stuff? I had to wonder if that was wise. I envisioned myself in a science fiction movie, all aglow with radiation and grotesque lumps growing all over my green skin, and perhaps a third eye. Then again, if I had cancer in my bones, better to find out sooner rather than later.

I returned for the scan a few hours later. The test took about 45 minutes, during which I lay on the table without movement while the scanner did its thing and the technicians did theirs. I was really getting the hang of stillness. I did it by letting my mind take me to the far away galaxies and earthly pleasures. I was on a beach, I was flying through fluffy white clouds, I was visiting loved ones.

Flights of fancy aside, there was no denying that I was flat on my back again, in a hospital again, and feeling vulnerable again. Every time I thought I was free of all this, it came back to get me. Michael Corleone and me. "Just when I thought I was out...they pull me back in."

I could see the monitor and the eerie outline of my own skeleton. I didn't know what to look for or what "normal" should look like on a full body bone scan, but the images didn't look good to me. I was pretty good at reading faces, but in this case, the technicians' faces were closed for business. I didn't catch That Look, but I still braced myself for bad news.

A visit with Dr. G a few days later proved me wrong. Both the bone scan and the X-ray were clear. They couldn't find a thing wrong with me.

My doctor explained that my coccyx could be sore due to the long car ride, or the fact that I had lost weight and my behind lacked enough padding. It could be a bruise or a hairline fracture too small to show up on the X-ray. It could be a lot of things, but it was not cancer and that's all I wanted to hear.

It turns out he wasn't really all that suspicious because

the coccyx would be a very unusual place for breast cancer to return. He just wanted us all to be sure.

The coccyx never did get better. Two years, several doctor attempts, and a special coccyx-friendly seat cushion later, it still hurts. Guess you just have to learn to live with some things. In the great scheme of things, a sporadic pain in the ass doesn't seem so bad.

CHAPTER 20

For the rest of your life, Babe

October 14 arrived, marking the one-year anniversary of The Day of the Lump. My own personal Lump Day. It was Breast Cancer Awareness month again and it was time for Pristine to get another mammogram. You and me both, Corleone.

I sat, waiting my turn for the inevitable paperwork that must accompany each medical procedure. I answered the same questions I answered the month before and fended off the shakedown for a check because I'd more than met my deductible and knew my insurance would cover it. Past experience told me that if you give in and write the check, it's not so easy to pry it back out of their hands after your insurance pays them, too. They tend to put overpayments on your account as a credit toward future expenses. Sign this. Sign that. Go back and wait.

I surveyed the room filled with women waiting for mammograms and other diagnostic tests. Were some like me...seasoned veterans who'd heard bad news? Were some first-timers, unsure what to expect? Some were nervous, of that I was certain.

I watched them enter through the double doors, one by one, as others exited through those same doors. The same doors I came through the previous October, knowing I'd be back for a biopsy the next day. The same doors that separated Jim and me when Dr. H and Stephanie exchanged That Look. Was "a" doctor back there?

Suddenly I was living in two time periods simultaneously,

as past and present collided in a rush of sights, sounds, and emotions hanging heavy in the air. *Please let it be different this time.*

My name was called and it was time to move forward. With only one breast to view, the process was faster. Then it was time to wait, with the gown still on, while Dr. H or a doctor I did not know studied the images of my left breast. Come on, Pristine, you're on the front lines and you've got to hold your position.

"You're good to go," the nurse said with a smile. Good to go. Nothing to see here, so move along. She handed me a rose, a Breast Cancer Awareness Month tradition, and sent me on my way, seemingly unaware of the enormous impact of her words.

It had been a year since my diagnosis and I'd aced a colonoscopy, a bone scan, and a mammogram. It was a triple play in my book, about as "cancer-free" as I would ever be.

After treatment ended, it was inevitable that people would ask the question. "Did you beat cancer? Is it all gone?"

With all the doctors on my case, none would say I was cancer-free, but one and all said that I should assume that I am...and on that day, I began to feel free of cancer's grip at last.

Whether or not some wayward cancer cells remained, awaiting the chance to spring into action, I could not know, but I didn't need to know. I had beaten it because it did not destroy me. Jim beat it, too, because he didn't let it destroy him – and together we beat it because we didn't let it destroy us. My kids beat it because they looked it straight in the face and carried on. My doctors and nurses beat it because they treated me as a fellow human being who needed their expertise and they did the best they could. I was still alive. We beat it in every way that mattered. True surviving.

Rose in hand, I walked through those double doors like an actress entering stage right to an up-tempo. No one looked up, but as I moved through the waiting area toward the lobby, I made a silent wish that all the other women present would have good results, too. I couldn't wait to get home and share the news with Jim.

For weeks, Jim had been working feverishly on getting the paperback version of *No More Secs!* published, making sure the cover design and page layout were just so. He took a photo of me holding the final proof, still wearing my little black cap to hide the very unattractive new hairdo forming underneath. On October 25, the physical book went on sale.

It's hard to find the words to describe the feeling of holding your own book in your hands. With cancer treatment behind me and my MS still in remission, my desire to see that book published had been fulfilled. It was out there for anyone who was interested, and each sale felt like a dream come true.

Readers shared their appreciation with me, adding to my elation. October 2011 turned out to be a very different story than October 2010, and for that I was – and still am – very grateful. Despite my misfortunate at having MS and cancer, I consider myself to be an extremely fortunate woman to have come so far.

There was a feeling of renewed energy and thoughts of what we would do next. It would be all too easy to fall into old patterns, saving the good stuff of life for later. It's good to plan for the future, but you have to live now, too. Nobody is guaranteed a long life – we're all subject to the uncertainty of it all. That's why we treat life like a household budget. It's wise to put something away for the future, but it's also important to live in the here and now.

For most women with breast cancer, initial treatment is followed up with five years of hormone therapy of some kind. These therapies greatly reduce the chances of recurrence, and according to the American Cancer Society, help patients live longer. For me and my triple-negative sisters of the world, hormone-based therapies are ineffective. Although I would be on a strict follow-up schedule, there was no more treatment on my horizon, barring a new recurrence. No pills or prescriptions. It was over.

After the end of treatment and the bone scan scare, it was time to reclaim control over my life, much as I did with MS. What kind of life did I want to live? Did I want a lot of follow-up testing to constantly reassure myself, or would life be more pleasant with a more relaxed approach? For Jim and me, the answer was clear. Absent any new signs or symptoms of cancer, I would visit my doctors at regular intervals, but we would not live our lives in fear, nor would we seek out medical tests without just cause. Of course, the MS could return and throw a wrench into those plans, but with my remission holding firm, it was easy to keep those thoughts on the back burner.

The future was wide open.

I sing and dance when I feel good. Not well, mind you, but I have a mighty fine time with it. I can't always say the same for those who must listen.

David was in the front seat, Liz and Tommy in the back. We were heading off to taekwondo class, as we did two or three times a week. Life with three little kids can be crazy busy and we spent an awful lot of time in the car on our way to one event or another. It seemed like a good time to crank up some Billy Joel tunes and let loose at the top of my lungs. I was just finding my groove when Tommy, still but a toddler, said, "Mom, can you please sing inside your head?" His honesty earned a laugh, and that about sums up my singing talent.

My singing is important, though. It's a sign that I feel good. It's not just a good mood thing – it means I feel healthy and have extra energy to burn – and that hasn't always been the case.

While preparing dinner one night I was in my usual fine

form, taking a stab at classic rock and belting out some fairly horrific sounding notes. Then I thought about Jim, working in our home office, and wondered if I was annoying him. How could he concentrate with my concert going at full volume? But it felt too good to stop.

Because of our experiences with cancer, he appreciates just about anything I do, simply because I'm here to do it. That's got to wear off eventually, right?

That night at dinner, I asked the question. "How long will it last? How long will I be able to get away with making a racket like that before you quit appreciating my mere presence and ask me to cut it out?"

Thoughtful pause.

"I'd say pretty much for the rest of your life, Babe. Sing all you want. I like to hear it."

Wow. There's not much more to say about that.

CHAPTER 21

A Promising New Chain of Events

We all get those odd emails that seem to be from people we know but are, in fact, spam. Shortly after Thanksgiving, I received one of those. It appeared to be from my sister, but it seemed to be soliciting me for a timeshare. That couldn't be, so I emailed Sis and asked her if she sent the email. She had.

Life takes some interesting turns. I had no idea at the time that the email in question was the first link of a promising new chain of events that would change the course of our lives.

Sis was acquainted with a woman who had a timeshare in Williamsburg, Virginia. She and her husband generally used it during the first week of December each year so they could enjoy the holiday festivities of Colonial Williamsburg. She wouldn't be able to use it that year because her daughter had recently been diagnosed with breast cancer, of all things, and they needed time to make important medical decisions. She was aware that Sis had a sister who lived in Virginia, and on such short notice, she figured we'd be able to use it.

That's not the kind of thing that happens very often in my life. Random gifts don't make a habit of falling into my lap. I hated the idea of such a young woman having breast cancer and hated the thought of benefiting in any way from their troubles. The woman was insistent. They couldn't use it and neither could anyone else. If we didn't use it, it would be wasted, and that would benefit no one.

After much discussion about neglecting work, we decided

to take her up on her offer. Instead of the seven days she offered, we would drive down on Friday and come home on Monday. Neither Jim nor I had been to Williamsburg, though it was only about 200 miles from our home base. What we would do there, we hadn't a clue, but we were eager for the adventure.

The drive went quickly, and our timeshare check-in went smoothly. In no time, we were unpacking our bags and familiarizing ourselves with our surroundings. Then there was the question of what to do. A myriad of brochures filled us in on activities in the historic triangle of Williamsburg, Jamestown, and Yorktown. The holiday season was in full swing, with parades, concerts, decorations galore, and endless attractions.

We decided to start out with a trip to Jamestown for a firsthand look at the original settlement site. The day was crisp and sunny, perfect for an outdoor adventure. I was glad I wore my sturdy boots and thick socks as we trudged through the winding trails. Our guide was in period dress and remained in character as he told of the hardships the settlers endured through the harsh winter. History came alive and I was grateful for the things that make modern life easier. A person with my health history would not have been able to survive under those conditions.

Next, we set out for Colonial Williamsburg. We parked at the visitor's center and began the long walk back in time, the walkway marking interesting points in history. The wooded trail was bustling with people, talking and laughing and generally enjoying the experience. Oh, how we walked that day!

Throughout our stay, walking was our main mode of transportation, me in my sturdy boots sans cane or need for a break. How different things were just a few years ago, when I had trouble walking the distance from my sofa to the kitchen. We continually marveled at my MS remission. Aside from the sparseness of hair, I looked as healthy as anybody else in town. Thank you, MS, for hanging back long enough for me to enjoy the physical pleasure of keeping up.

For a small city, Williamsburg offers an abundance of restaurants, from super casual to fine dining. We would not go hungry.

Over lunch one day, we took advantage of a large window to watch passersby. It wasn't cold enough for snow, but there was a foamy bubble machine going and children were playing, running under the bubbles and catching them as best they could while pretending it was snow. The atmosphere was lively and we found ourselves caught up in the mood.

At an Italian restaurant one evening, we finished our pizza and one of us, I don't remember which, said out loud what we were both thinking. Williamsburg should be on the short list. The short list being the list of places we'd like to live. Choosing that place wasn't easy, due to the fact that our children and extended families were scattered around the country. There was no home base for us. There was no one place that we could call home or where the bulk of our family lived in close proximity.

Through my health problems, we'd come to realize one very important thing about moving. It would put my health insurance at risk. In most states, it would be impossible for me to get insurance. Period. In a handful of states, I'd have access to some coverage, but little or no choice regarding the type of plan and whether or not it would cover my pre-existing conditions.

Worse than that, potential insurers couldn't or wouldn't talk specifics unless we actually moved to their state. They couldn't promise that any plan we discussed would be available, and they couldn't offer quotes with any degree of certainty unless we were 30 days or less from a move date. How are you supposed to relocate without knowing whether or not you'll be able to have health insurance?

All that was scheduled to change with the Affordable Care Act, but until that thing was in full swing, these were risks we simply could not afford to take. The political scene being what it is, we couldn't count on it actually taking effect or remaining in effect in 2014 and beyond. While my health insurance was a huge financial burden, at least I had it, and with my health history, it would be folly to put it in jeopardy.

That's why the short list was so short. Pretty much every location on it had been scratched off over the years. The new short list was a Virginia-only list, since as long as I could afford to pay for it, I could keep the one and only policy available to me in my state. It is what it is.

Williamsburg is a very small city, but it has a vibrant downtown. The sprawling campus of The College of William and Mary attracts the young population and other amenities attract families and retirees. Visit the downtown area any day of the week and you'll find people from all walks of life strolling about or dining on outdoor patios.

More than any of those obvious things, we noticed something else. It's not a thing so much as a feeling. You know what I mean. It's that "X" factor that you can't quite describe. The intangibles of time and place that let you know, in your gut, that you fit in.

The combination of northern evergreens and lush tropical vegetation heightened my senses, reminding me that I am part of the earth and a tiny part of a much bigger picture.

As our little adventure came to a close, we knew we'd revisit Williamsburg, either as a weekend getaway, or as something more.

CHAPTER 22

Happy New Year

The calendar was about to turn from 2011 to 2012. Normally, I don't give much thought to the new year. Oh, it's a fun excuse for a party, but I never got particularly excited about the event itself. It's just another day. There was yesterday, there's today, and there's tomorrow. Every day. What's in a number?

Except that the turning of the calendar page that year was something I wasn't sure I'd see in good health – or at all. But there I was, in all my glory, making my awkward dance moves in public amidst the streamers and balloons.

Several glasses of wine and the pulsating music helped pushed me over the edge into I-don't-care-what-I-look-like-I'm-having-a-good-time mode. I was wearing a cap, with a second paper Happy New Year hat on top, and dancing with an attitude. It was soon going to be 2012 and I was there to see the transition.

Laissez les bon temps rouler!

Without warning, an overwhelming feeling of euphoria began to well up, coming from the far recesses of my being. It began at my toes, flowing upward throughout my entire body and spirit, growing more powerful with each passing minute. It went to my head made me feel at one with my body and the universe.

Life!

My enthusiasm was spiraling out of control. I was jumping and cheering and laughing on the dance floor, raising my hands high above my head as I danced. I was aware of more than a few curious stares, but also a lot of smiles in acknowledgement of my celebration. Those who glanced in my direction seemed to understand my jubilation. If they didn't, I didn't care.

I was alive! Really, and truly alive! In a matter of minutes, it would be 2012 and I would be there. I'd live to watch my children blossom, to write more books, and to expand my horizons. I'd be there to share it all with Jim.

Ten...nine...eight...

My watery eyes must have made it appear that I was crying, but that couldn't have been further from the truth. I was laughing, inside and out.

Seven...six...five...

The room was exploding with anticipation and excitement, everyone gearing up for the big moment.

Four...three...two...

Cue the music!

One! Happy New Year!

Balloons and confetti fell over us like fluffy snowflakes. At least I imagined balloons and confetti falling from above. It may have been all in my head. No matter; it's the spirit of the thing that counts.

Jim whirled me around and with a gentle touch, planted a sweet kiss on my lips, a simple, brief act that encompassed so much more than anyone else could possibly understand. It told a tale of love and the promise of more to come.

We raised our glasses, sipped our champagne, and proceeded to hug those closest to us. We danced a little more before the band packed up, and when the 1:00 a.m. breakfast buffet arrived, we settled down and filled our bellies with our first meal of the bright, shiny new year.

Little did we know just then how much our lives would change before we turned the page on calendar again. The year 2012 would be a bittersweet year, bringing both great sadness and a promising new beginning.

For as long as I could remember, I had naturally straight, thick hair. Then came cancer and chemotherapy and the bald head that goes along with that. I didn't mind my bald head because I had more important things to ponder.

When it began to grow back in such haphazard fashion – multi-colored and multi-textured, I didn't mind that either because, without eyebrows and eyelashes, it was obvious what I'd been through. I had an excuse for my appearance.

By the middle January, it was time to give up the hats and begin familiarizing myself with this new and somewhat embarrassing mop. I didn't look like a cancer patient anymore. I gained a pound or two and there was some color in my cheeks. Suddenly I realized that I just looked like a person with BIG, weird hair. It was thicker than ever, but bore little resemblance to *my* hair. Curly in the back, straight around the front, and ridiculously frizzy all over. I finally understood that whole humidity/frizzy hair thing. I would have been the height of fashion in the big hair days of the 80s. Of course, back in the 80s, I actually permed my hair to get that look. Yeah, it's life's sense of humor at work again.

So engrained was my self-image, that I startled myself each time I passed a mirror. Alas, none of the fussing or torture I put it through could beat the beast into submission. This new crop had a mind of its own.

During a moment of quiet reflection, it finally dawned on me. There are life lessons in my hair.

Life is all about change. It's a journey that waits for no one. Without change, we would stagnate. Ready or not, want it or not, change does come, and sometimes it's for the better. If not, we must learn to adjust.

Being a little different is a blessing, not a curse. When we're young, we strive to fit in. We try to dress, act, and speak like our peers. As we mature, we embrace those things that set us apart. "Unique" is a compliment, not an insult, at least in my book.

To swim against the tide is courageous. To attempt to reverse the tide is futile. You have to pick your battles. Pick those that truly matter. My hair. It tells my story...and I think I like it.

On a related note, there's another little thing about cancer survivors I'd like to share. Those of us who lost hair through chemotherapy understand how completely insignificant hair is in the great scheme of things, we really do. We know, with every fiber of our being, that it is better to be alive with goofy hair or no hair than not to have survived at all.

If we talk about our hair, please don't think you have to remind us how fortunate we are to be alive. We don't need reminding, thank you. We are NOT comparing hair to life. If we happen to mention that we're having a bad hair day, take that as a healthy sign. It means we're not consumed with thoughts of cancer or treatment or death. That's a good thing.

We can have a bad hair day just like everybody else, so let us have this admittedly trivial, but very human, everyday moment.

CHAPTER 23

Cancer Returns, but it's not what you think

The next few months passed quietly, as we settled into life After Cancer. I was mindful of the warnings I received about depression or anxiety following cancer treatment, but those emotions never came.

Perhaps that was because I was pleasantly engrossed in my work. I was promoting the book and my regular clients were keeping me busy. I was beginning to make notes about a work of fiction I'd been kicking around. It would be a challenge, to be sure, but one I relished. I always wanted to write fiction.

As a young girl, I often begged my sister for the opportunity to borrow her portable Brother typewriter, even though I didn't know how to type. I adored the sound it made as keys clanked against the paper and roller, the energetic little "ding" as you reached the end of a line, and the swoosh of the carriage return. I even liked the eraser with the brush on the end. I wanted to put my fingers on the home row and form words. I wanted to see those words fill a whole sheet of paper. I wanted to write something for others to read.

I don't know where I got the image, but it was probably from those old black and white movies that took place in noisy newsrooms. I fancied myself a Katharine Hepburn-like character, sitting in a smoke-filled room, a pencil behind my ear, piles of crumpled paper all around, pounding away at my latest novel. I was a weird kid.

Decades later when I finally sat down to write a book, it

wasn't a novel, but a memoir. There was no smoke-filled room, no pencil, no piles of crumpled paper, and typewriters were just a bit of nostalgia. But I pounded away on a laptop in my home office, at the kitchen table, and on the living room sofa. And I do mean pound; I type hard. You can hear me going at it from a great distance. I pounded away for a year and a half before producing the first draft of *No More Secs!*

I no longer fantasize about that smoke-filled room because, well, I hate smoke. I haven't written that novel yet, either, but there's no doubt about it, my childhood fantasy came true.

In April, cancer reared its ugly head once more, but I was not its host. Seemingly out of the clear blue, Jim's 84-year-old father was diagnosed with an advanced type of cancer that was impossible to treat. His age, combined with other health problems, meant that the best we could hope for was to help him live as comfortably and as pain-free as possible for as long as possible. A few months, at best, we were told.

It was a totally different experience than my cancer. I stood a good chance of living a long and fairly healthy life after aggressive treatment. In Dad's case, there was no question about the eventual outcome. There was nothing to be done, and Dad didn't want to do anything, anyway.

For me, it was very sad news. For Jim, it was an attack of epic proportions aimed squarely on his family. Cancer again. Cancer was shadowing him around like a twisted stalker who gets his kicks by letting you live, but striking the people you love the most.

The drive from our home to Dad's took about five hours, but we had to get up there to see him. It was an emotional roller coaster.

Jim's Dad was a doctor, a general practitioner who spent his lifetime healing others. He knew exactly what he was up against. After his diagnosis, he was ready to walk out of that hospital for good. He wanted nothing more than to go home and sit in his familiar chair and enjoy the love of his wife, family, and friends. And he did just that.

In May, Jim and I were scheduled to participate in our local Walk MS. I'd been fundraising for a while and there really wasn't any reason to cancel, but it was hard to focus on the event. The walk was held in a magnificent park on one of the most gorgeous spring days ever.

The participants and volunteers were all focused on MS, while we were distracted by cancer.

It was a day in which all manner of emotion – sadness, grief, gratefulness, appreciation, and fear – rattled around in our consciousness. The funds we raised went to the National MS Society, a big contributor to research into the cause of and treatment for MS. In most previous years, I needed a cane and had to take the walk very slowly. Once I even needed a wheelchair to get through it.

In 2012, however, I walked entirely on my own leg power and at a good pace, too. My MS had been in remission for two years and I'd been through treatment for triple-negative breast cancer. In the meantime, my father-in-law was in his final months of life, a life he would soon lose to our mutual enemy.

The walk was about five miles long, and Jim and I were each lost in our own thoughts about MS and cancer and life and death and hope and sadness. It was a physically invigorating, but emotionally exhausting walk. No sooner did our feet cross the finish line than we hightailed it out of there. We didn't care about the snacks or the drinks or the music. We weren't interested in socializing. We just wanted to go home.

Our lives turned into a series of whirlwind road trips. Back and forth we went, from Virginia to New Jersey and back again, each time knowing that this trip might be the last time we'd see him alive. There were health care decisions to be made, arrangements to make, and a constant vigil by family, friends, and caregivers.

Dad took his leave in early June, quietly and in his own home. The good doctor, who had helped so many others in his lifetime, was gone from this world. It was my second twinge of survivor's guilt.

I lost my own father a long time ago, but that didn't prepare me for the emotions I felt as I witnessed Jim writing a eulogy for his, or for the painful lump that formed in my throat as he read that heartfelt eulogy in front of the assembled mourners, many of whom dabbed their eyes as he spoke.

Throughout those difficult months, the harsh reality of cancer, and the speed at which it can do its work could not be ignored. There's Before Cancer and After Cancer, it's true, but After Cancer world isn't free of cancer. Just because I don't have cancer, doesn't mean it can't come into our personal space. It had, once again, changed everything.

CHAPTER 24

The Wisdom of Bees

Spring turned to summer and we fell into a comfortable routine. Though I no longer looked like a cancer patient, the emotional toll of Dad's cancer once again laid our emotions bare. The many road trips during his illness took a toll as well, and we were on a self-imposed road trip break. It was Jim and Smokey and I, just doing our thing, but something was nagging away at us a bit.

What's next?

What about that move we always talked about? Our house was a comfortable size, but the yard work was becoming too much and threatened to get away from us. It was more space than we needed, of that there was no question.

Jim and I don't care for clutter and we don't buy things just for the sake of having them. I, in particular, tend to get a high from getting rid of things. The more clear space around me, the better. It actually makes me feel anxious when I'm in an overstuffed home.

Outside of the house, there was something else we had that we could probably spare. My 11-year-old car was still in very good shape. The only problems it had stemmed from the fact that it wasn't getting much use.

After I left my job at the funeral home, there were great stretches of time during which my car was hardly used at all. Since we both worked at home and generally went everywhere together, it was easy to acknowledge that we should be a one-car family. Still, it wasn't an easy decision.

On the pro side, getting rid of the car meant substantial savings on state property taxes, auto insurance, and upkeep. On the con side, well, a one-car family has less flexibility. We'd have to keep our schedules coordinated. There's a certain level of uncertainty and vulnerability that comes with not having your wheels available at all times and having no back up vehicle.

The thing that finally sealed the deal was when I went out to my car one day to discover that my little bee friends were back. Apparently, they were in the middle of a building boom. They were simultaneously constructing new homesteads behind the passenger door mirror, inside the rear door, and in two exclusive, highly desirable locations in the trunk. My car was prime real estate.

The bees knew. They knew before we did that it was time to make a change. They'd been trying to tell me all along that I was hanging on to something I no longer needed and their message was finally sinking in. The car represented an idea, a lifestyle that was no longer relevant, or perhaps it was a lifestyle that I thought I should have.

Okay, my little bee friends. It's not going to make you happy, but I'm going to take your advice.

I'm not a car person. I don't know the first thing about makes or models or prices or horsepower. For me, cars are about transportation. If they're comfortable, nice-looking, and get the job done, that's enough for me. But the car and I had been together for over a decade, and I felt a slight tug of emotion as we discussed the pros and cons of letting it go.

The truth was, we didn't need two cars anymore, and if our situation should change, we could always get another car. That was it. Time to let go and give that one-car-family thing a try.

Jim served the bees with their final eviction notice, had the car professionally cleaned, and readied it for sale. By the following weekend, the deed was done. We took the first step toward a simpler, downsized life. There comes a time when you must stop the daydreaming and take action. If you don't take a step forward, you're never going to make your dreams come true.

Change was in the air. Was it my cancer or Dad's or something else altogether that stirred things up? The events of the previous year and a half were swirling around us like a tornado that, rather than moving on, hovered in place. The only remedy for that was to jump into the twister and take it for a ride.

CHAPTER 25

Lights Out

Each day, we received real estate listings by email. We signed up for multiple email blasts years ago, and just kept adding and subtracting locations as we played with our short list. Some locations were there just for the fun of daydreaming. We knew we'd never move to Key West, but even if you're never going to live in a beach house, it's fun to look.

It was a normal afternoon, both of us working in the home office, when Jim let out a "hmmm..." He'd just spotted a listing for a condo for sale in Williamsburg.

"Take a look at this," he said, pointing to the screen. I wheeled my chair closer as he scrolled through the pictures of the inside, then the outside of the condo.

"It's cute." We poured over the details – the square footage, amenities, and number of bedrooms and bathrooms. It was in our price range.

"I'm going to call this realtor," he said. "We liked Williamsburg a lot. It can't hurt to talk to her."

He must have felt fairly inspired to actually make the call. Or itching for change. Or at a loss for what to do next. No matter, I felt the same way.

He placed the call and put it on speaker. We spent a half hour chatting with the realtor. She was talkative, and it turned out she was originally from New Jersey, so she and Jim hit it off instantly. Before he hung up the phone, we had committed to driving down on Saturday to take a look at the unit from the ad, plus two other units in the same condominium. It's funny how a decision is years in the making, then seems spontaneous when it finally comes to fruition.

After we hung up the phone, we looked at each other as if to say, "What were we thinking?"

Were we really going to drive 200 miles just to look at properties in a place we barely knew anything about? Yeah, that sounds just about right for us.

We got more than we bargained for when we hit Williamsburg – and I mean that in the nicest way. We toured the property and the individual units that were for sale.

One was bank owned and in need of some major work. The second needed a major facelift, but was located in the back of the building, so it boasted more privacy and offered a green view from every window. The third was in much better condition, but located in the front. It would provide less privacy and a less attractive view of the parking lot.

A big consideration was whether or not we wanted a home with two levels. We always said that if we were to move, we'd need a single-level home. When my MS was raging, stairs proved to be a significant problem. Once you have MS, you never stop thinking about alternative methods of getting things done.

Despite the long remission, we were keenly aware that my MS could return, and if it did, those stairs might as well be Mt. Everest. However, the condo units were set up with a master bedroom on the main floor as well as on the upper level. The only other thing in the upper level was the loft, which would function as our office.

If either of us ever had difficulty maneuvering the stairs, we could always move to the downstairs bedroom. Wireless Internet meant we could work from anywhere in the house. Also, the stairs were a straight shot up with no curves, so installing an electric seat lift was not entirely out of the question. We decided it was a workable situation.

Overall, we were pleased with what we saw, but our realtor guide didn't leave it at that. When she realized how little we knew about the area, she decided to do something about it. She drove us around the city, pointing out restaurants, shops, and other things we hadn't yet discovered.

A few years before, we vacationed at Virginia Beach and loved it. It even made the short list, and it was only 60 miles away from Williamsburg. One hour from the beach? It's not quite a beach house, but we were getting closer.

What we didn't know until that day was that Yorktown is home to a hidden gem of a beach. The small, but charming area is right out of a picture postcard. Locals walking barefoot, shoes in hand; families spread out on blankets under colorful beach umbrellas; children splashing in the water; boats in the distance. Motorcycles lined the street in front of the local pub and shoppers drifted around the quaint little shops. Tourists were snapping photos of historical points of interest and stopping to enjoy ice cream cones. And all that was a mere 16 miles from the condo.

It was as if our realtor contracted with a theater company to set the scene for would-be buyers.

We again sensed that…je ne sais quoi…that elusive feeling of place. All in all, it was an enlightening day.

After dinner, we were ready to head back home. As soon as we were alone in the car, we began to discuss the details of the day. We veered right into details of the individual units, as though moving to the area was a foregone conclusion and we only had to decide which unit we wanted.

We dismissed the bank-owned property right away, although it was priced to sell. We weren't interested in taking on the renovation required, or dealing with the red tape. I was particularly intrigued by the back unit with the green views, but we finally settled in on the more move-in ready unit.

The decision was both impulsive and well thought out, if that makes any sense. A combination of things over a two-year span pushed us into taking action. These weren't things we discussed on a daily basis, but things that swirled around just below the surface, a reminder of precious life and our limited time on earth.

Before we made it a hundred miles out of town, we decided we were going to place an offer. Before we made it two hundred miles, the realtor called to ask how we felt about the day. We told her which unit interested us most and that we'd most likely be placing an offer, but we wanted to sleep on it overnight.

That we did. We slept on it, woke up on it, discussed it over breakfast, and placed an offer. We set the wheels in motion. Just like that, life was going to change again, only this time it was by choice.

The counter offer came within a few days and left us with a reasonable place to meet. Upon making that offer, we were told that the owner decided not to sell after all. Well, now, that was unexpected and disappointing. Was it a sign? If so, we chose to ignore it. We weren't about to let a thing like that stop the forward momentum.

After more discussion, we placed an offer on the other unit. It seemed to me, that although it needed some sprucing up, it had the three things a piece of property should have – location, location, and location. I knew we would enjoy the outside view from the back of the building and in the end, that place would be in our best long-term interests.

A few weeks of back and forth negotiations and the deal was set. We scheduled closing for two months out, figuring that would give us plenty of time to get our current home on the market and plan the big move. We really were going to do this thing!

We quickly set things into motion on the other end. We made an appointment with our realtor friend and started talking about how best to ready our house for market.

On the last Friday in June, the temperature soared well into the high 90s. We intended to spend the weekend sprucing the place up, but Mother Nature had some input into the matter. In the early evening hours, a fierce summer storm swept into the area, knocking out our power and our forward momentum.

We did the things you do when the power goes out. We dug out our flashlights, lit a few candles, and got ready for bed, hoping the evening air wouldn't be too stifling without the air conditioner. It was stifling, of course, but the power would surely be on in the morning, or so we thought.

The morning light revealed quite a bit of wind damage. Small to medium sized tree limbs were sprinkled around our yard and the surrounding yards.

Attempts to reach the power company resulted in long hold times and recorded messages. It didn't look too promising. There was only one road leading into and out of our neighborhood, so after we dressed, we decided to take a walk to survey the situation.

Downed trees and a power line running straight across the road forced cars to pass in the narrow section that was still clear. There was no sign of a work crew and we knew it was going to be a long, hot, sticky day.

Jim made the rounds of our yard, stacking tree limbs, branches, and twigs in a neat pile on the side of the house. There are few things I hate more than wasted food, and the contents of our recently stocked refrigerator were spoiled. Even though sunshine provided a lot of light, we were not up to the task of cleaning, painting, or staging anything because the thermometer was dancing around the 100-degree mark again.

We did some reading, played cards at our bistro table on the deck, and generally frittered the day away. Our energetic plans were broken and we were at a loss for what to do with ourselves. Even Smokey looked as though she might wither away.

By late Sunday afternoon, we were losing it big time. Heat, humidity, and frustration were growing. Just when you think you're moving forward, you spend three days sitting around sweating.

We didn't care what movies were playing, but decided that a few hours in a movie theater would provide a welcome relief. As Jim carefully maneuvered the car out of our neighborhood, we observed that nothing had changed since the storm. The trees hadn't been touched and the wires were still hanging precariously over the street. One wire crossed under the paths of cars and there was still no sign of a crew of any kind.

With a neighborhood full of kids, that couldn't be good. We knew there was a lot of damage and many people without power throughout the area, but since this was our neighborhood's only access road, we figured we'd waited long enough.

Jim pulled out his cell phone and made one more forceful plea to the powers that be, noting the possibility of justifiable anger if that wire injured someone, especially a child.

I don't recall what movie we saw, but I do remember how good it felt to sit through it. We went to one of those movie theaters where you can eat a meal while you watch. We generally don't like to make a meal out of that type of food, but home cooking was not an option and sometimes you just have to compromise.

After the movie, as we turned the corner onto our access road, we saw a crew hard at work, setting up a temporary system of wires that would remove the safety hazard and get our electricity running again. Hallelujah! The weekend was coming to a close, but at least we could start Monday morning off with the comfort of modern conveniences.

We rescheduled the appointment with our realtor and planned to begin staging the house on Monday. We meant business. We were determined to let nothing derail the plan.

CHAPTER 26

A Downsized Life

As anyone who has ever listed a house for sale knows, it's a trying experience. You fix it up, you make appointments, you wait while strangers examine your home, and you do it all over again. When you work from home, it disrupts the entire workday. You wonder if you're properly showcasing the home's positive features and if you're priced right. And you keep cleaning and tidying and staging. It's takes constant attention to detail.

Even though we hadn't yet received a genuine offer by September, the condo closing was on the schedule and it was time to take care of that end.

We prepared for the drive by filling the Subaru with as much as it could handle. Cleaning supplies, a couple of folding chairs, a card table, some basic kitchen necessities, an inflatable mattress, and various odds and ends made the first cut. It was all so exciting!

The closing went off without a hitch and we walked out with a set of house keys. The occasion lacked some of the usual excitement associated with buying a new home, since we weren't actually going to move in. It was thrilling and scary as hell at the same time. For awhile, at least, we would be dual homeowners, something we sincerely hoped would be a temporary insanity.

We surveyed our new home, hardly believing we actually did this thing. It would require a much bigger facelift than we realized before, but we were primed to enjoy the process.

I've never been camping. I don't like sleeping bags and I don't have any desire to share the night with insects or other creepy crawly things. Our inflatable mattress is about as close I want to get to roughing it.

The mattress was queen sized and we had an electric inflator, the right sized sheets, and our favorite pillows. It wasn't uncomfortable, but it did prompt a lot of tossing and turning, and it made noise with every movement. It was interesting; I'll give it that. At least we didn't have to worry about being eaten by bears.

"Let's have a pajama party!" We arranged blankets and pillows on the floor and surrounded ourselves with board games, video games I didn't understand and could not hope to conquer, and all manner of food and drink. It was a ritual, something we did to break routine every now and then. We'd spend the whole night together, the kids and I, acting rather silly and fighting sleep. Sometimes it was a fort or a ship at sea or a bunker. Always, it was a good time.

We spent the weekend cleaning...and cleaning...and buying more cleaning supplies...and cleaning. No matter what we had to do on the inside, there was little to be done on the outside. That's the part of condo life we would come to appreciate in short order. A little puttering was to be expected, but there would be no more backbreaking yard work.

I have a thing about buildings, especially homes. I think they hold onto the emotions created within their walls. I base this on nothing scientific; it's just a feeling I get when I enter a building.

This particular condo had a chaotic feeling. It was unsettled and cranky. One of the first things we wanted to change was the paint color in the kitchen. All the walls were painted red — not a cheerful shade of red – an angry shade of purplish red that made it feel as though the walls were closing in on us. Combined with an oversized black refrigerator and light fixtures that reminded one of tarantulas that could reach out and touch you at any moment, it was not conducive to the sense of calm we desired.

We're a harmonious couple, but we found ourselves at odds in that kitchen, breaking out into uncharacteristic bickering, and that was totally unacceptable.

We walked around each room, discussing the color scheme and the all-important placement of furniture. It sounds like a trivial matter, but where you place your furniture has everything to do with how well your home will function and how you'll feel within it. We wanted to create an easy flow, much like we had in the other house.

When two people work at home full time, flow and function are of the utmost importance. Do it wrong, and there's no escape. Night and day, that's your world. We needed to do it right so our constant togetherness would continue to work for us, not against us. Fortunately, it was a process we both enjoyed.

After a busy weekend getting to know our new home, we locked the doors and headed to our other home, which had the potential to become an albatross if it didn't sell soon.

Offers weren't rolling in. What a pain in the you know what. We're very neat and clean, anyway, but it was still difficult to maintain that "buy me" look. That's because we weren't only moving – we were downsizing.

My car, thanks to my bee friends, was only the first step. We also had to go through all our possessions to decide what was worth keeping and what wasn't. Things had to go. We placed ads and sold a few large items, and we gave some others away to acquaintances, but the main beneficiary of our downsized life was our local Goodwill Store.

As I packed our less important things for the move, I also packed boxes full of items we would donate. I once had a collection of books to rival a small library, but that would no longer do. We donated hundreds of books we knew we'd never read again. Farewell, old friends.

I'd long since gotten over the whole "real" books versus e-books debate. It's a false choice and not an either/or question. If it's reading that's important to you, it shouldn't matter if you read something electronically or off paper or off the wall of a cave. And once you pass the hurdle of believing you must keep books just for the sake of keeping them, it's very freeing. Downsizing your personal library doesn't mean you have to give up reading or that you can't hang on to some favorite books.

I think "stuff" is an anchor. Things begin to feel like responsibility and added weight. When you buy a condo that has nice, roomy closets, but no basement or garage and no attic storage to speak of, you have to be organized. Luckily, I like to organize. I actually get a kick out of trying to make things fit in such a way that you can keep the things you want and get to them whenever you want. I could probably have a good career as an organizer.

Jim and I have a rule. Every time something new comes into the house, something else must go. You'd be surprised how well that system works. The best thing about downsizing is that the things you decide to keep, and the things you decide to buy, tend to be of high value. That is, you take your time in making purchasing decisions and you choose better things because you aren't wasting your money on things that have no importance.

When you go through a major illness or live with any type of chronic illness, simple living means less time spent on chores and more time being productive or having a good time. Just by being alive, we've all got stress. We can't get rid of all the stress in our lives, but we can get rid of a lot of self-imposed stress. An uncluttered living style creates a peaceful, easy vibe.

As the weeks passed, we continued to go back and forth between the houses, each time loading up the car with kitchen tools and things we didn't want to leave to the movers.

All the activity and anticipation pushed health concerns

to the back of our consciousness. Other than the normal aches and pains of midlife and the pain in my coccyx, there was no reason to worry about health. If either MS or cancer were going to reappear, it wouldn't be able to stop the momentum created by our move.

Breast Cancer Awareness Month was rolling around again, and so was my scheduled mammogram. For some reason I felt a slight trepidation that my run of good fortune was about to end. Things were going well – we were actually moving – and the last time things were going that well, I was diagnosed with cancer. Just my luck to have it happen again.

I was another year removed from cancer, but it hit me like a ton of bricks the second I entered the place. I suppose there will always be things that remind me of those difficult days, and perhaps that's a good thing.

The process went as smoothly as always. I accepted my pink rose, along with good news, and walked back through those double doors and into the outer waiting room, my footsteps as light as my mood.

October is the month I was born; it is Breast Cancer Awareness Month; it is the month I was diagnosed with breast cancer; it is the anniversary of my survival. It is a good month and my pleasure was evident in the blog post I wrote to express my appreciation:

> "I am two years old today. Sort of. Two years ago today, I learned for certain that I had cancer. I remember that conversation as clearly as if it happened yesterday. "It's very serious," said my doctor. "Things are going to move very quickly now. You've got a tough fight ahead of you."

> "He wasn't wrong about any of that. Triple-negative breast cancer is a force to be reckoned with, and we went after it with a vengeance. Triple-negative breast cancer is more aggressive than other types of

breast cancer; there are fewer treatment options, and it is more likely to recur during the first five years after diagnosis. That's why I'm glad I didn't wait to get that suspicious lump checked out, and that's why I'm celebrating my second birthday today. Actually, that's why I celebrate just about every day.

"When the American Cancer Society talks about candles on the birthday cake, I know what they mean. It's not about pink ribbons or "ta-tas" or any of the other superficial fluff that goes along with breast cancer talk. It's about life and death.

"Earlier this month I quietly celebrated my 53rd birthday and today I lightheartedly celebrate turning two years old. Here's to you, Life. Lucky, lucky me."

With plans for the move and a house on the market, whole days passed wherein I didn't think about MS or cancer, even in a fleeting way. Life was happening and we were part of it.

CHAPTER 27

Sold! Sort of

With a price drop, we suddenly found ourselves with several potential buyers, which eventually led to a contract. In an emotional sense, it was exactly the contract we wanted. It was with a lovely young couple with a baby on the way. This was a couple who could make use of the spacious backyard and roomy basement we barely used. They would inject new life into the home we'd grown to love, and that would make it easier to part ways.

In a financial sense, it was acceptable, but less than ideal. The couple planned to use a USDA-backed mortgage, which meant that it could be several months before finalization. A new waiting game was underway.

Just as we did for so many events in our lives, we acknowledged the worst-case scenario – that the loan would fall through and we'd have to start all over again in a few months. Then we moved ahead in the hope of the best-case scenario – that the loan would go through and the sale would be complete before Christmas.

A tentative closing date was set for early December and we continued our back and forth life, sprucing up the new and packing up the old.

We ripped out the old, pet-damaged carpeting and replaced it with beautiful dark hardwoods. We thought long and hard about colors, and contracted with a painter who could complete the work before our move.

Meanwhile we continued purging our possessions and

packing boxes in the hope that the sale wouldn't fall through.

The focal point of our living room was an enormous copper-look planter that held a lovely palm tree. The large planter was also home to a smaller planter, a ceramic dog, and a small water fountain. To the casual observer, it appeared that the water fountain was part of the planter.

We kept the water fountain running all day, adding a lovely background sound and providing Smokey with her main water source.

The planter and the tree were actually left to us by the previous owners of the house because it was too awkward to move. We added the fountain and other accessories and it soon became an oasis in our living room.

I couldn't imagine not transferring our little oasis to our new home, but the measuring tape insisted that there was no good place for it. We offered it to our buyers, but they didn't want to give up the space, and I couldn't blame them, what with a baby on the way.

So, I packed up the water fountain and smaller plants and repotted the tree into a smaller, lighter pot. I scooped the dirt out of the enormous planter and Jim carried it outside by the bucketful. At last, it was empty and I could give it a good cleaning.

We gave the huge pot away to a man who bought our kitchen table and chairs. He seemed rather pleased with the freebie and said it would look great on his oversized front porch. Of that, I have no doubt.

It's strange, the things that prompt emotion, but I knew I would miss that old pot and my little oasis.

I've relocated before, but it turns out that leaving doctors who helped you get through cancer is not so easy, especially so soon after the end of treatment. I set appointments with my surgeon and my oncologist. I wanted one final visit with each, to make sure I was tiptop and to express my gratitude. I entrusted my life to these doctors and they honored that trust. If cancer returned, I wouldn't have my familiar team to spring into action. I'd have to take my chances with someone new, and that was an unsettling feeling. I had to let go of that security blanket.

Whether or not cancer returned, I still needed to visit with a doctor every six months until I reached the five-year mark. Fortunately, my oncologist was able to recommend someone in Williamsburg so there would be no break in my care.

While all this was going on, Smokey was getting herself out of sorts. She didn't appreciate strangers entering the house while it was on the market and she certainly didn't like the boxes. The sound of a box being assembled or packing tape being pulled would send her scurrying for cover. Her insecurities were building by the day, and insecure cats can be quite a handful.

We were all ready to leave the chaos behind and wrap it up.

By the first week of December, we learned of a delay in the closing. It would likely be put off until January. It was an uncomfortable delay, as we didn't want to be living out of boxes for the holidays, and the buyers were anticipating a New Year's baby. Everyone's plans hinged on everyone else's and we were all at the mercy of the USDA. With a government shutdown looming at the end of the year, we were concerned with the many ways it could affect all of us.

Jim and I decided to move anyway. We were going to throw caution to the wind and take our chances. If the deal fell through, it would become a royal pain. We'd have to list the house again, even if it was empty. We set a moving date for the second week in December and set the wheels in motion. Que sera, sera.

By that time, we were well into the era of After Cancer when I was supposedly at risk for anxiety or depression. Still, it didn't happen. I believe there are two contributing factors that helped me avoid it.

First, our lives didn't change all that much during treatment. Our work and play routine remained basically the same, just at a bit of a slower pace.

Second, although the decision to make a major life change on the heels of our family's cancer double-whammy may have appeared a bit rash, it was a good decision. Our high level of activity and focus on achieving a goal put most thoughts of recurrence behind us. We finished treatment and smoothly transitioned back into our lives.

I guess that would be my advice to the newly diagnosed. Keep on doing what you do and stay on track with your goals.

CHAPTER 28

The Sweet Spot

Moving day is one of the great bittersweet occasions of life. No matter what your reasons for leaving, you're leaving a piece of yourself behind, along with your sense of home and all that is familiar.

It's not quite as difficult when you put yourself in the shoes of previous generations. Those who left a homeland to conquer new worlds and those who left a family behind to settle far away knew they'd probably never see or speak to their families again. Now, that was rough.

These days, we have cell phones, texting, social media, video chats, and all manner of transportation. Even when we leave a place, we're always within reach.

The movers came in on a Wednesday morning and spent all day carefully wrapping our furniture, protecting the floor, and loading up the truck. We weren't sure we'd actually purged enough. Some things we brought with us just in case we could make them work. We were secure in the knowledge that there was a Goodwill on the other end, too.

Our things would be stored overnight on the truck and the movers would set out for Williamsburg early the next morning. We, on the other hand, figured we'd better get Smokey settled in on the other side. We took everything else with us, except for a few cleaning supplies for our return visit at closing.

After a long day of movers coming in and out and kicking up a racket, Smokey was beside herself with fright. She wanted to curl herself up into a tiny ball and disappear. She didn't even want Jim or me to touch her. Past experience told us that she would hate the car ride. Just going to a veterinary appointment 10 minutes away was enough to set off a bloodcurdling cacophony. It was going to be a long, uncomfortable ride.

It was dark when we finally arrived at the Sweet Spot, so named for a variety of reasons. I always wanted a home with a name, and this one struck a cord. It's a combination of things that makes the name Sweet Spot a fitting one.

Back when we were working on our short list, we thought about weather and seasons. Jim, being from New Jersey and I, from Rhode Island, are both partial to a four-season climate. On the other hand, he spent a few years in the hot, humid climate of New Orleans and I spent many a winter in the frigid northwest suburbs of Chicago. We were not fond of extremes. Southern Virginia offers four very distinct seasons that unfold slowly so each can be enjoyed. To be sure, July and August would be very hot and humid, but it seemed to us to be a suitable four-season climate.

Another thing that was important to us was its proximity to transportation. Not too far to hop on a train or a plane; not too far off main highways. We added about 90 minutes to a road trip to visit family in any direction, but nothing's perfect.

Like life itself, the Sweet Spot fulfilled most of our needs, but not all of our desires, and that was good enough for us. The important thing was that we were not going to keep waiting for the right time to move. Waiting for the perfect time is what can keep you from ever taking that next step.

One of Jim's daughters sent us a housewarming gift. It was a clock with the words "Sweet Spot" on it. The name would stick.

As exciting as it was for us, Smokey was in no mood for all the commotion. She came out of her travel cage in a state of discombobulation and wanted only to find a safe place to hide.

The three of us spent a restless night on the noisy inflatable mattress. The next day promised to be a big one.

The movers must have set out well before dawn because they showed up before 9:00 a.m. Smokey, who hadn't eaten or had a drink of water since we arrived, would need a safe place to hide. We took her water and food dishes, along with her litter box, and left her in the upstairs bathroom, safe from the movers she so feared.

Unfortunately, she would not be able to escape the sounds of the men carrying large pieces of furniture and boxes. Her trauma continued from within the confines of the bathroom, where she steadfastly refused food and drink.

Most people consider moving day to be one of life's more stressful events, but aside from fretting about Smokey, I wasn't feeling any stress. I couldn't wait for the movers to finish their work so we could get started unpacking and organizing ourselves. I was in full-on nesting mode, eager to start setting up housekeeping.

The move represented many things, not the least of which was the fact that I was alive to do it. It was a fresh start and everything felt fresh and new. The future was wide open, welcoming us with open arms.

When the movers were finished with their work, we invited Smokey to come out and have a look around, but she was having none of it. She slunk away into the downstairs bathroom, figured out how to open the vanity, and crawled inside. There she stayed for the better part of two days, immune to coaxing. She wouldn't be sold on the Sweet Spot for a few more days.

Jim's priority was to set up our home office in the loft. He arranged our desks and got to work setting up the all-important electronics so we could continue to work and respond to our clients' needs.

Over the next few days we unpacked, stacked cardboard boxes, and decided what items still needed to be purged. We briefly toyed with the idea of not bothering with Christmas decorations, but once again, we could not resist. We were in our new home for Christmas and it should look like it.

We moved the treasured palm tree from one room to another in an effort to find the perfect spot. Meanwhile, the water fountain that was part of our everyday lives was not living up to its former reputation. The acoustics of the condo turned what was once a pleasant background sound to a noisy distraction in our new home. C'est la vie. Out it went.

Our Christmas gift was word that our buyers' USDA loan went through and an official closing date was set for January 4, when we could finally end the drawn-out moving process and settle down in our one and only home.

By what miracle was I enjoying the physical hustle and bustle of moving during the holiday season? How was it possible that this 50-something-year-old woman with MS was not only functioning, but also thriving? That I cannot answer. One thing is certain – time is precious and should never be squandered. We were making the most of it.

CHAPTER 29

Ignore the Omens

We drove back to the old homestead on the morning before closing so we'd have plenty of time to give it a good cleaning. We wanted the young couple to come in knowing they'd made the right move. With their baby expected to enter the world any day, we knew they were probably frantic at the thought of all the work involved in moving. We wanted to start them off with a positive feeling. We wanted them to get as much out of the house as we had.

The place was empty except for our trusty inflatable mattress and some cleaning supplies, but the peaceful, easy feeling we loved so much remained.

The front door was made of thick wood and stained a rich, dark brown. Instead of a little peephole, it had a small working door through which you might be expected to provide a password before entering a speakeasy. It welcomed visitors with a large lion's head door knocker. Now that's a door with character. I would miss that door.

Within those walls was the imprint of our lives. We could still feel the emotions swirling around as we cleaned and inspected every detail.

The kitchen, in particular, held so many memories. It truly was the heart of our home. It's where we'd linger after dinner, talking and laughing over a glass of wine.

It was in the living room where I could picture the family sitting with us on the weekend before my surgery, where we passed the pleasant evenings all cozy and warm, and where we put the Christmas tree every year. We once put a 2,000-piece jigsaw puzzle together in the dining room. That little home office is where I cranked out my very first paid writing. The house was alive with warm memories and it felt good to be handing it off, like a good luck charm, to a growing family.

We visited the backyard where Smokey's brother, Bandit, was laid to rest and would remain, and I took one last look at the faded birdhouses Tommy and I painted together years before.

We said goodbye to our neighbors, a wonderful couple who used to peek in on the cats for us when we weren't home. It was the house in which we started our business, and where we lived, laughed, and loved our way through MS and cancer. It was the house where we mourned losses and celebrated triumphs.

We would leave the home behind on its green plot of land in its all-American neighborhood, but the memories would always be part of the history of us.

Later, we would learn that the new owners moved in immediately following the closing and brought their new baby girl into the world later that same night. They were off to a great start. New memories were already forming within those walls.

Finally free and clear of our obligation to that house, we immediately headed back to Williamsburg, eager to celebrate and begin anew. It was the first week of January, and the weather was clear and crisp, as if we ordered it up special for the 200-mile drive.

I'm not really big on omens, but that short journey seemed to be telling us something. Only an hour into the drive, we found ourselves stuck behind a large truck with a full load of precariously stacked oversized logs. It was not hard to imagine the impact one of those huge logs would have if it let go. I still shudder at the thought. The jam-packed highway made it difficult to maneuver into another lane, but Jim finally found his moment and we both felt better for it.

But wait, what's this? The driver of the car in front of us was weaving slightly out of his lane to left, then slightly out of his lane to the right, first speeding up, then slowing down. We really needed to find a way around this guy before something bad happened, and it took another long while before we were finally able to shake him.

About 20 minutes later, another large truck worked its way in front of us and, as it did so, a huge chunk of ice broke free from the roof, blasting through the air and slamming into the windshield right in front of Jim's face.

The startling cracking sound made us both duck and flinch, but Jim recovered quickly and kept us on track. In an amazing bit of good fortune, the windshield didn't actually crack.

We looked at each other, mouths agape. Our day started off really well, but it seemed we were on a path with danger. We just wanted to make it back to the Sweet Spot in one piece. Or we could look at it another way. Maybe the universe was working to keep us safe because we did make it home, none the worse for wear, and a little lighter for the elimination of a big budget item.

There would be no more back and forth, no more packing and unpacking, no more inflatable bed, no more decisions about what to keep or where the major pieces of furniture would go. It was all coming together nicely.

Smokey was comfortable in her new surroundings at last. She delighted in perching at the top of the staircase like a lioness overseeing her territory. We set up a convenient window seat for her so she could hang around in the office with us and still see outside. She would spend most of her days there, acting as our office mascot.

We spent the rest of the weekend on the finishing touches, putting every little thing in its place, and I do mean every little thing.

Jim and I, left unchecked, can be a bit...well, too detailed. Jim went about the task of hanging each and every painting and photograph so they were exactly the same height at center. Really.

As we had with our previous home, we wanted our new condo to have a clean, fresh feeling. I organized the closets, drawers, and cabinets to the nth degree.

We were down to minutiae. Perhaps that chair would look better if we moved it one inch to the right. Seriously. We got that carried away with our quest for the right feel, especially where the office was concerned, but it was all in good fun.

We were very serious about getting things back on track. When you work from home, having an organized, comfortable environment is everything, and we were all set. We went to bed that Sunday night feeling very accomplished. With the focus on our home out of the way, we made a pact that come Monday morning, we'd be at our desks bright and early, ready to focus on our work.

The previous two years took a heavy toll. After dealing with my cancer, Dad's cancer, his death, living in a home that was on the market, and preparing for the move, we'd lost countless hours of productive work time – and we needed to rectify that. It was time to set things right.

It was a brand new year and it was our hope that the Sweet Spot would help us take it on.

It felt good to be home.

CHAPTER 30

Oh, and then there's *that* look

We took our seats shortly before 9:00 a.m. on a beautiful, crisp Monday morning. Smokey took her place on the bench in front of the window, basking in the early sunlight.

The new year lay before us full of promise and we were ready to take it up a notch. We settled in at our tidy new desks, feeling as fresh as a couple of kids on the first day of school.

Jim quickly busied himself with a web project while I tackled an article that was due that afternoon. As is often the case, we each became so absorbed in our own tasks that the morning passed by with barely a spoken word. That's what it's like when you work inside your own heads.

When my stomach began to rumble loud enough for Jim to hear, I decided to head down to the kitchen to scrounge around for lunch.

I felt at one with my new kitchen. The formerly offensive walls were painted pleasant shades of cream and green. "Hearts of palm" it was called, and it helped bring the great outdoors in. The room was small, but open to the main dining area and sunroom. We still planned on replacing the over-bearing light fixtures, but other than that, we'd transformed it into a space we could enjoy, and I was doing just that.

I picked up the coffee carafe and our two coffee mugs from earlier in the morning, setting them in the sink. Might as well wash them before taking on lunch, I thought. We still washed dishes by hand for the most part, even though we had a dishwasher. Washing dishes is a good opportunity for me to let my mind wander freely. In our new kitchen, it was also an opportunity to gaze out of the large windows of the sunroom. Such a beautiful day.

I turned on the hot water and squirted some dish soap into the carafe. There was a sound of running water coming from above, and I assumed Jim was using the upstairs bathroom.

When the carafe was cleaned and rinsed, I reached for a coffee mug. Hmmm...I could still hear the water from above. It sounded as though a small river was running over my head.

I turned off the faucet and listened again. That's when it hit me. Jim took a shower hours earlier, so there was no way he was using the shower again. Something wasn't right.

"Hon!" I called. "Are you running water upstairs?"

"I thought you were...what the...?!"

There was a great commotion from above as Jim sprang into action. I ran up the stairs, two at a time, toward the bathroom. Jim was on the floor with his head under the sink.

Water was shooting upward from behind the faucet handle, and streaming down the mirrors and walls. Water was pouring out from underneath the vanity, our toiletries floating like little ships at sea.

Water covered most of the bathroom floor and was rapidly spilling onto the bedroom carpeting, into the closet, and out into the hallway between the bedroom and loft.

Jim was working frantically to turn off the water. "It's broken! I can't turn it off!"

"The main!" we shouted in unison.

We raced back downstairs toward the laundry closet off the kitchen. Jim grabbed the handle of the water main, turning with all his might, until at last our water supply was cut off.

Our eyes turned upward toward the freshly painted kitchen ceiling. A dark circle was growing wider by the second and a hole was forming a few inches away from the light fixture.

Even though the main was off, the river of water was still flowing between the upstairs floor and the downstairs ceiling. The sickening sound of rushing water continued as it began to find its way down through the cranky old light fixture and onto our brand new hardwood flooring.

Jim reached for the large garbage can, using it to catch the flow, while I dug out an old vinyl tablecloth to protect the floor. Small pieces of ceiling began to crumble.

It only took about four minutes for the mini disaster to unfold, but it played out like a slow motion movie scene.

We must have looked like those cartoon characters that run off the edge of a cliff but don't realize it until they look down. For one brief moment in time, we stood frozen in disbelief. We turned toward each other and our eyes locked.

There's that look again. Well, not That Look, but it was a look, all right.

AFTERWORD

After watching Ann write two memoirs over the course of the past five or so years I can only say that it's about time she let me put in my two cents. Seriously – thanks, Babe. And while I'm no expert in these matters, I'm going to nonetheless address my comments to those who have been stricken by diseases like cancer, as well as to their families and caregivers, oftentimes one and the same.

I suppose there are other diseases just as bad, but cancer has a way of initiating profound core changes in those who come into contact with it. For the afflicted, there's often a physical change that must be endured. As with Ann, parts of your body are taken from you in an attempt by your doctors to stop the assault. But it goes well beyond the physical. Other change is more intangible... internal... metaphysical if you will. When you're dealing with cancer, EVERYTHING else in life takes a backseat to your fight for survival. You begin to seriously ponder the not-so-far-fetched notion that in a very short time you may cease to exist. You sit at night to eat with your family and try to picture the scene when you're gone. The touch of your partner is tinged with sadness as you both try to imprint the feel of each other in your brains; memories stored for the days when physical touch is no longer possible. Your partner may not say it, but they can't help but wonder what it's going to feel like eating alone, sleeping alone, thinking of something funny or interesting to say, but not having anyone there to laugh or comment.

Yep, cancer truly sucks and there's really not a whole lot I can say to make you feel good about it.

There are many different kinds of cancer. As humans, we tend to slip them into neat categories as we think their names. Breast cancer, colon cancer, lung cancer, liver cancer, pancreatic cancer, prostate cancer, brain cancer, ad infinitum. They all add up to one thing. Life's never going to be the same. Your assumptions about life and all you think you know up until your doctor broke the news of your cancer's existence to you are about to be tested.

This isn't conjecture. We went through this and, while I'm sure that everyone's cancer experience is not quite the same, I can only write from personal experience. You see, Ann and I have learned to roll with the punches. And that, my friend, is what I recommend you do, too. If you've got cancer and you're looking for the reason why you got it, here it is -- shit happens. It's that simple. Roll of the dice and all that rot. It's what you do after you find out you've got it that really matters.

Do you roll up in a ball and wait to die like some tend to do? Maybe. In fact, sometimes, once you hear the details, you can't really blame some people for doing just that. That's a bit harsh, but remember, we must be honest with ourselves if we're to get through this. The truth is that while we're all going to eventually die, most of us think about our own death in some far off terms. It's something that will probably happen to us sometime way way WAY in the future. And while we should acknowledge that a diagnosis of cancer really is sometimes a death sentence, the good news is that more often these days it is not.

Sometimes a cancer diagnosis is a bit more like a really big, really loud wake-up call. And as far as I'm concerned, whether you've got three months, three years, or a pre-cancer expected lifetime ahead of you, it's always a good thing if you listen when a life buzzer sounds. It means that it's time to put down everything and take stock of your life. With cancer, it means that now is your time to make a decision.

Fight or flight? What do you do when your enemy is at the gate? Do you cut and run, or do you fight? Ann decided to fight. And I decided to fight right along with her -- for her, for me, for our kids, for us. That doesn't mean we sat around just thinking positive thoughts, hoping the effort would solve our problems. That's just stupid. Cancer doesn't care if you're happy. By the time you've got it, cancer also doesn't care if you decide to start eating healthy, or exercising, or any other such thing. You probably should have been doing those things all along. But it is OK to start now. You are your own army and an army needs to be well fed.

Ann and I decided to fight. We were the generals in our little army and we oversaw a small batallion of experts: doctors who we trusted with Ann's very life. Our weapons had really scary names: chemotherapy, mastectomy, radiation, and others that I can't even pronounce. We put our trust in science, prayed to our God for luck, listened to and questioned our doctors, took ownership of the situation and made it a point, each and every day, to make sure that our partner was still OK. That meant taking time out for ourselves, and for each other. We made it clear to everyone... work, family, friends... everyone... that getting through this ordeal was our top priority. We would do anything, spend anything, go anywhere to make that happen.

In the end, we were lucky. We won. At least, we think we won. Cancer could be watching and laughing as I write these words, knowing it plans to strike again. There are no guarantees, so we've never asked for any. But we know that if the worst does happen that we will each reach down and fight again. Like the book says, there's always time to live, to laugh, and to love. Until there is time no more.

I hope this is the last memoir that Ann ever needs to write in the "Living, Laughing & Loving" series. I hope she can put her mind and her talents to work writing a work of fiction, or any other thing that makes her happy. But if life decides that it wants to pick on our little family once again, then life should know that we're ready for it and that we will do what we always do. We will fight.

I hope that each of you decides to do likewise.

With love,
Jim Pietrangelo

A Word From the Triple Negative Breast Cancer Foundation

- Triple-negative breast cancer (TNBC) is one of many forms of breast cancer.
- 15-20 percent of all breast cancer cases are classified as TNBC.
- Forms of breast cancer are generally diagnosed based on the presence or absence of three "receptors" known to fuel most breast cancer tumors: estrogen, progesterone, and HER2-neu.
- A diagnosis of TNBC means that the tumor in question is estrogen-receptor negative, progesterone-receptor negative, and HER2-negative. In other words, TNBC tumors do not exhibit any of the three known receptors.
- Receptor-targeting therapies have fueled tremendous recent advances in the fight against breast cancer. Unfortunately, there is no such targeted therapy for triple-negative breast cancer.
- TNBC tends to be more aggressive, more likely to recur, and more difficult to treat because there is no targeted treatment.
- TNBC disproportionately strikes younger women, women of African, Latina, or Caribbean descent, and those with BRCA1 mutations.

Triple Negative Breast Cancer Foundation
PO Box 204
Norwood, New Jersey 07648
(646) 942-0204
tnbcfoundation.org

ACKNOWLEDGEMENTS

I'm forever grateful to my family for their love and support, especially my husband, Jim, and my children, David, Liz, and Tommy. I love you.

In the interest of privacy, I refer to my doctors by initial only. My sincere appreciation goes out to them and the other medical professionals who saw me through my cancer treatment. I'm so very blessed to have found doctors who have both knowledge and compassion.

To all the strangers and acquaintances who reached out with words of comfort, I cannot begin to describe the power behind your thoughtfulness. Words do matter.

Many thanks to my writer friend, Steven B. Williams, author of *Her Mother's Eyes* and *Heartsnare*. Nothing like a fellow writer to kick your ass at the exact moment when your ass needs kicking. (Or "arse," as Steve would say.) I do kick back, though.

My heartfelt thanks to Diane Radford, MD, FACS, FRCSEd. She has been a wonderful source when I'm writing articles about breast cancer. It is truly an honor to include her foreword in this book.

A tip of the hat to the dedicated staff and volunteers of Beyond Boobs!, an organization I discovered when I moved to Williamsburg, Virginia. Beyond Boobs! supports young women diagnosed with breast cancer and provides breast health education for all. I'm very pleased to play a small part in their mission of helping others. Learn more at beyondboobs.org.

Special thanks goes out to the Triple Negative Breast Cancer Foundation for their valuable input.

Writing is a lot more rewarding when you have readers, so thank you, too.

CREDITS

The cover of this book was designed and created by Web-Camp One, LLC using artwork from the following sources:

Dancers: cd123 / 123RF Stock Photo
Red Tear: christopherhall / 123RF Stock Photo
Woman's Eyes / shygypsy / Shutterstock

www.ingramcontent.com/pod-product-compliance
Lightning Source LLC
Chambersburg PA
CBHW060453290526
45791CB00001B/100

ABOUT THE AUTHOR

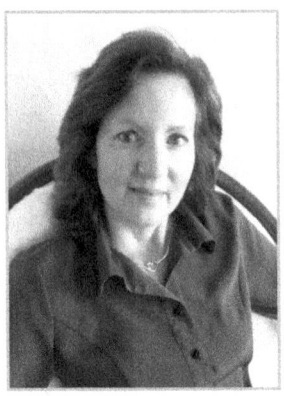

Ann Pietrangelo is a freelance writer and a member of the American Society of Journalists and Authors. She and her husband, Jim, are partners in WebCamp One, LLC, a full-service website development and content creation company. They're living, laughing, and loving in Williamsburg, Virginia.

AnnPietrangelo.com | WebCampOne.com
Email: writer@WebCampOne.com

Also by Ann Pietrangelo
No More Secs! Living, Laughing & Loving Despite Multiple Sclerosis
Website: NoMoreSecs.com

Spread the word! Online reviews help readers discover new books. Now that you've read *Catch That Look*, please consider giving a quick review on Amazon, Goodreads, Barnes & Noble, or other book sites. It is sincerely appreciated.